पुरातत्त्व
पुरातत्त्व
PURĀTATTVA

Bulletin of the Indian Archaeological Society

No. 21 1990-91

Editor
K. N. Dikshit

Jt. Editor
B.R. Mani

D.K. Printworld (P) Ltd.
New Delhi

Cataloging in Publication Data — DK
[Courtesy : D.K. Agencies (P) Ltd. <docinfo@dkagencies.com>]

Purātattva : bulletin of the Indian Archaeological Society, no. 21, 1990-91 / editor, K.N. Dikshit ; jt. editor, B.R. Mani.
p. cm.
Includes bibliographical references.
ISBN 8124602964

1. Archaeology — India — Periodicals. 2. India — Antiquities — Periodicals. 3. India — Civilization — Periodicals. I. Dikshit, K.N. II. Indian Archaeological Society.

First Published in 1991
First Reprinted in 2005
ISBN 81-246-0296-4
Price for volume 21 (1990-91): Rs. 800 US $ 40

Reprint authorised by
Indian Archaeological Society
New Delhi - 110 016

Purātattva is published annually.

Manuscripts (whether in the form of articles or notes or book reviews) offered for publication should be sent to the Editor, Purātattva, Indian Archaeological Society, B-17, Qutab Institutional Area, New Delhi - 110 016.

Published and printed by:
D.K. Printworld (P) Ltd.
'Srikunj,' F-52, Bali Nagar
New Delhi – 110015
Phone : (011) 2545 3975, 2546 6019 Fax : (011) 2546 5926
E-mail : dkprintworld@vsnl.net
www. dkprintworld.com

PURATATTVA

CONTENTS

Editorial

ARTICLES — PAGES

1. Early Representations of Buddha and Buddhist Traditions in Aśokāvadāna — 1
   M.C. Joshi
2. The Role of Computer in Archaeology — 7
   Aparna Sengupta
3. The Legacy of Indus Civilization in North India — 17
   K.N. Dikshit
4. Excavations at Karkabhat — 21
   A.K. Sharma
5. Inscribed Copper Tablets from Mohenjo-daro: Some Observations — 25
   B.M. Pande
6. Benginning of Iron Age in Garhwal, mid-central Himalaya: An Ecological overview — 29
   Vinod Nautiyal, K.P. Nautiyal, B.M. Khanduri, D.L. Rajput
7. Ceramics and Maritime Routes of India: New Evidence — 37
   I.K. Sarma
8. Identification of Setavyā, the Ancient City of Kosala with Siswania and its Terracotta Art — 43
   B.R. Mani
9. Role of the Individual's Perception and Important Explanatory Modes in Archaeology — 51
   Vijneshu Mohan
10. The Lady of the Beasts or The Lord of the Beasts: A Reappraisal — 57
    P.V. Pathak
11. Defence System in Ancient India based on Literary and Archaeological Evidence — 65
    V.C. Sharma

NOTES AND NEWS

12. Deceipherment of Script by Soviet Scholars — 71
    Hem Chandra Pandey
13. Anangpur - The Palaeolithic site near Delhi — 73
    A.K. Sharma & S.B. Ota
14. Excavations at Golabai Sasan, District Puri, Orissa — 74
    B.K. Sinha
15. Khaparkhera: A Submergible Chalcolithic Site — 76
    S.B. Ota

16. Excavations at Ladyura, Almora, U.P. 77
A.K. Sharma
17. Harappa Horned Deity: The Evidence from Padri in Western India 79
Vasant Shinde
18. Identificaiton of Pundravardhana 81
Achyutanand Jha
19. Discovery of an early Inscription from Pitalkhora 84
S.K. Mittra
20. Role of Temples in Medieval Orissa 85
K.P. Padhy
21. The Northern Black Polished and Other Associated Wares from Ropar 87
K.C. Nauriyal
22. Rock Engravings at Tabo, Distt. Lahul and Spiti, Himachal Pradesh 90
A.K. Sinha
23. Report on the Chemical Analyses of the Glasses from Khairadih 92
Ravindra N. Singh & A.A. Abdurajakov
24. Analytical Investigation of Indian Bronzes 96
M. Singh
25. World Archaeological Congress 99

BOOK REVIEWS

26. M.L. Varadpande. Mahabharata in Performance 103
C. Mani
27. Anatoly I Martynov. The Ancient Art of Northern Asia 104
K.N. Sikshit
28. D. Guillanme. Analysis of Reasonings in Archaeology 105
D.P. Agrawal
29. B.R. Mani. The Kushan Civilization 105
K.N. Dikshit
30. Gopal Narayan Bahura and Chandramani Singh 106
Catalogue of Historical Documents in Kapad-Dwara, Jaipur, Part II
P.K. Trivedi
31. V.R. Mani. Sons of Siva A Study in the Religious cults of Ganeśa and Kārthikeya. 106
Amarendra Nath
32. Lallanji gopal. The Economic Life of Northern India C.A.D. 700-1200 107
Y.B. Singh.
33. Urmila Sant. Neolithic Settlement Pattern of North-Eastern and Northern India 107
K.N. Dikshit
34. Prakash Sinha, Model for Land-use in Late Acheulian Tradition (Satna District, M.P.) 108
K.N. Dikshit

PURATATTVA

Number 21 1990-91

Editorial

This is the twenty first issue of Puratattva, a Bulletin of the Indian Archaeological Society. It introduces the readers to numerous recently discovered archaeological sites in India. There are both macro and micro studies, field surveys and latest thoughts on some old issues. This issue will hence be of interest not only to archaeologists but to cultural anthropologists, art historians, epigraphists and others. In a situation where archaeological discoveries are fairly large, we shall be failing in our duty, if we do not acknowledge the cooperation received from Sh. M.C. Joshi, Director General, A.S.I., who has allowed the members of the Survey to publish their material in this issue. All the illustrations, be they Line drawings or Plates are by the courtesy of the institutions to which respective contributors belong. We are also thankful for the substantial financial support extended by the Archaeological Survey and Chairman, Indian Council of Historical Research in bringing out this issue. We also express our thanks to Prof. C. Mani of Mussoorie for help and to Shri Manish Chandra of Punjab Printing Press in the speedy publishing of this journal.

We may also inform here that the Government of India has agreed to host the forthcoming World Archaeological Congress (WAC-3) in 1994. A note by Prof. Jack Golson, President, World Archeological Congress, may be seen by our readers.

Early Representations of Buddha and the Buddhist Traditions in Āśokāvadāna

M.C. JOSHI*

Buddha or Jina as a concept indicating the highest development of man in the form of an 'Enlightened Being' was possibly already known before the time of Śākya-muni Buddha. Yet it is certain that there was hardly any tradition to suggest his presence through specific forms, motifs or symbols for the purpose of propitiation or worship. India and Srilankan traditional accounts (Sharma 1984: 14) about creation of Budha's portrait during his own life time and later have hardly any historical substance and these appear to be late inventions to justify the creation of Gautama Buddha's representation in anthropormorphic form during subsequent periods.

The internal evidence preserved in early Pali literature recording an observation of Buddha (Gautama) in this regard clarifies the issue pertaining to worship of his relics in precise terms.

According to *Mahāparinibbāna Sutta,* Buddha, just before his death, told Ānanda not to bother to worship his mortal relics *(sarīra)* after he is no more but should only attempt to achieve the essence of Dhamma. The *Sutta,* however, further records that the Blessed One knew that his intensely devoted followers amongst knowledgeable Kshatriyas, Brāhmaṇas and Gṛhapatis would (certainly) offer worship to his corporal remains after his Parinibbāna. What was predicted by Buddha came true as all the eight *stūpas* built on his mortal remains by different groups in fact became objects of worship. In the third century Aṣoka as mentioned in the *Divyāvadāna* (Vaidya 1959: 240-41) exposed most of these old *stūpas* to obtain the original mortal remains *(dhātus)* of Buddha for redepositing them in numerous newly raised *stūpas,* stated to be 84000 in number, in different parts of his empire to popularize Buddhism in a much wider area than before. Evidence also shows that Aśoka attempted to formalize the form of the *stūpa* by decorating it with *chhatra, harmikā* and *vedikā* or railing.

A question emerges as to why the system of worshipping the *stūpas* containing sacred *dhātus* became popular despite the fact that Buddha himself did not favour the idea? What appears to be likely is that the Buddhists followed the popular belief based on age old tradition of sympathetic magic that any part or fragment of a man's body even either its detachment from the original form or its transformation continues to maintain inseparable relation with the original personality of person to whom it belonged once. It is on this account Buddha's mortal remains which were deposited, dug and redeposited in *stūpas* many a time were believed to represent his physical and eternal presence through the *stūpa* where it was desposited. This is also confirmed by the Buddhist traditions recorded in a later text like *Saddharmapuṇḍarīka Sūtra,* a Sanskrit text, compiled not later than the third century A.D.

According to an event narrated in this text, once Mahāpratibhāvāna Bodhisattva, enquired from Buddha about the significance of the mystical appearance of a *stūpa.* The Lord (Bhagavān), thereupon, replied to him that in this *stūpa* exists the actual body of one substance of a Tathāgata (Dutta 1953: XIII). The Gilgit manuscript also supports a similar idea referring to the presence of Buddha in a *stūpa* (Dutta 1953: XIV).

'अहं च दृष्टो इह शासनास्मि भगवांश्चयोयं स्थित स्तूप मध्ये।'

* Archaeological Survey of India, Janpath, New Delhi.

The attempt to provide a *chhatra* or *chhatrāvali* on the top of the *stūpa* also confirms the same idea that *stūpas* with relics were built to serve as lasting symbols of living Buddha or other great Buddhist monks. The *vedikā* provided it a specific structural personality like that of the *chaitya-vṛksha* which invariably represented a divine spirit.

Emperor Aśoka seems to have introduced some new symbols to represent Buddha and events connected with his life. From this standpoint, the most impressive example is his pillar at Sarnath with its lion capital, originally, supporting a *dharma-chakra* which not only gave it the character of a *chakradhvaja,* but also symbolized the Buddha delivering his first sermon at Mṛgadāva (pl. I). The four lions supporting the wheel served only as pedestal or throne in conformity with the ideal of *chakravartin.* This is also confirmed by a Bharhut relief where similar pillar with *chakra* at top has in its capital figures of deer and not the lions. In a Sanchi sculpture, the deer are depicted just below the pillar (pls. II and III).

Perhaps, Aśoka himself was responsible for inventing the concept of this memorial pillar, for it was also he who introduced many kinds of spectacles for the propagation of *dharma* in terms of dramatic performances, thereby, turning the *bherī-ghosa* (announcement for holding dramatic visuals) to *dharma-ghosa* (propagation of the law) (Joshi 1989: 16). His fourth Rock Edict expresses these shows more precisely as: *Vimāna-dasanāhasti-dasanā agikhandāni-cha-añāni diyvāni rupāi dasayiptā* i.e. views of celestial mansions or cars, celestial elephants, columns *(skandha* or *skambha)* of light and other divine forms (were arranged to be shown by Priyadarśin, the Beloved of the gods). Many of these divine spectacles find expression in the post-Mauryan art especially in early Buddhist architecture the *sudharma devasabhā* (celestial hall) in Bharhut rail (Pl. IV); divine elephant in depiction of Māyā's dream (pl. V) or elsewhere as a symbolic representation of Bodhisattva (Pl. VI) and flaming pillar in Amaravati sculpture (Pl. VII) or Chakradhvaja symbolizing Buddha expounding Dharma at Mṛgadāva in Sanchi and Bharhut reliefs. A notable symbol not mentioned in Aśokan edict under reference is, however, the Buddha-pāda or foot-print of Buddha which is used in the early Buddhist art especially that of Amaravati to indicate the invisible presence of the Master. In fact, this is the first attempt to depict Buddha in human form through the carved impression of feet (Pl. VIII).

Due to socio-cultural and other reasons, by about the beginning of Christian era and more vigorously in the subsequent centuries, the growth of Buddhism underwent a process of change, philosophically and artistically. These changes were mainly responsible for the innovation and popularization of Buddha depiction in human form and modification in the corresponding aspects of the faith.

The origin of Buddha's sculpture in human form itself is a much debated subject. There are scholars who feel that it originated in Gandhāra while others suggest Mathura as the place of its origin. In our view, the production of Buddha's figure in human form, in these two distant areas, appears to have been attempted almost simultanously and independently, without any conceptual borrowings from each other. But, what seems to be certain is that the idea to have an image of humanized Buddha, had the sectarian support of a section probably of the Sarvāstivāda school of Buddhism.

In this connection, we propose to draw the attention of art historians to some data associated with this subject in *Aśokāvadāna,* an early Sanskrit text of Sarvāstivāda origin which is vitally significant to understand the measures taken to justify creation of the anthropomorphic image of Buddha and popularization of its worship. The material under reference is preserved in *Paṁśupradānāvadāna* (Episode of the Gift of Dust), which itself is a part of *Aśokāvadāna,* (Vaidya 1959: 216 ff; Mukhopadhyaya 1963: 1 ff) and seems to have been composed in Mathura itself as it is basically connected with that town and its famous Buddhist monk Upagupta, believed to be a contemporary of Aśoka.

What is important for us in this Avadāna is the story of Upagupta who is stated to have converted Aśoka to Buddhism. According to the text, Upagupta was youngest child of a Gandhika (scent-dealer) named Gupta in the city of Mathura. He was ordained into Buddhism by a learned monk named Sthavira Sānakavāsī and he attained *arhatva* (stage of an *arhat)* in a short period. He was so important as a monk that he has been styled as a Buddha without *lakshaṇas (alakshaṇako-Buddha).* His birth at Mathura was stated to have been predicted by no less a person than Buddha himself when the latter visited the town of Mathura.

Upagupta is also said to have subjugated Māra like the founder of Buddhism. The details of the main part of the episode are described in the text as under:

One day when Upagupta was preaching the Law amidst a great gathering in the city of Mathura, Māra, the god of Temptation, showered strings of pearls amongst the assembled people to divert their attention. As a result, none could realize the Truth. Next day too, during his discourse there was again a rain of gold and real pearls. Upagupta's preaching remained effectless. On the third day when Upagupta began to expound the Dharma, Māra caused celestial damsels to appear there and to sing and dance with the playing of divine instruments. Consequently, the audience felt attracted towards the heavenly nymphs and their celestial music. Māra was delighted at this sight and placed a flower-garland around the head of Sthavira Upagupta. Thereupon, the great monk thought of subjugating Māra and created a flower garland out of the skeletons of a snake, a dog and a man. The garland was put around the head of Māra who on wearing it found that instead of garland there were skeletons of snake, dog and man tied to his head, neck and ears. Māra tried to remove the bones from his body but did not succeed. He then flew up into the sky and sought the help of the gods like Indra, Rudra, Vishṇu (Upendra), Yama, Varuṇa and other divinities, but they expressed their helplessness in the matter. Lastly, for his relief, he approached Brahmā who advised him to resort to Upagupta to quickly attain the deliverance. Māra then realized the greatness of Buddha as expressed in the following verses:

अथ मारस्तथागतशिष्यसामर्थ्यमुपलभ्य चिन्तयामास —
ब्रह्णा पूज्यते यस्य शिष्याणामपि शासनम।
तस्य बुद्धस्य सामर्थ्यं प्रमातुं को नु शक्नुयात।। २६।।
कर्तुकामोऽभविष्यत्कां शिष्टिं स मम सुव्रतः।
यां नाकरिष्यत्क्षान्त्या तु तेनाहमनुरक्षितः।। २७।।

किं बहुना ?

अद्यावैमि मुनेर्महाकरुणतां तस्यातिमैत्र्यात्मनः
सर्वोपद्रवविप्रमुक्तमनसश्चामीकराद्विद्युतेः।
मोहान्धेन हि तत्र स मया तैस्तैर्नयैः स्वेदित-
स्तेनाहं च तथापि नाम बलिना नैवाप्रियं श्रावितः।। २८।।

i.e. "Māra, having seen that a disciple of Tathāgata is more powerful than Brahmā, the god of creation, expressed his respect in the following terms: 'Who could measure the power of Buddha? If he wanted to vent His anger on me, what could He not do? It was His piety that the Great Compassionate One, did not vent His anger on me. It is only today that I know Tathāgata, the Great, Perfect, Compassionate One, the Great Fulfilled Benevolent One, who has attained the true deliverance. The ignorance blinded me. In all the places, I molested Him. Nevertheless, the Benevolent Buddha, the Compassionate and the Righteous One, never addressed me harsh words".

Consequently, with a feeling of deep repentance, Māra prostrated at the feet of Venerable Upagupta and requested for the removal of the skeletal fetters from his body. The great Monk agreed to do so on the conditions that thereafter Māra would not disturb the Bhikshus and he would also show to Upagupta the human form of Buddha, as the monk had seen only *dharmakāya* (body of essence) of Buddha and not his *rūpakāya* (physical form).

धर्मकायो मया तस्य दृष्टस्त्रैलोक्यनाथस्य।
काञ्चनादिनिभस्तस्य न दृष्टो रुपकायो मे[१४]।।
तदनुपममनुग्रहं प्रति[१८] त्वमिह विदर्शय बुद्धविग्रहं।
प्रियमधिकमतो हि नास्ति मे दशबलरुपकुतूहलो हाहं।।

Māra agreed to obey the commands of Upagupta to assume the form of Buddha but warned the Monk that he would not pay any respect to the God of Temptation (Māra) in his form as Buddha, for that would destroy (burn) him as he has no powers (capacity) to accept the homage which is actually intended for Buddha:

सहसा तमिहोद्वीक्ष्य बुद्धनेपथ्यधारिणम्।
न प्रणामस्त्वया कार्यः सर्वज्ञगुणगौरवात्।। ४०।।

बुद्धानुस्मृतिपेशलेन मनसा पूजां यदि त्वं मयि
स्वल्पामप्युपदर्शयिष्यसि विभो दग्धो भविष्याम्यहम्।
का शक्तिर्मम वीतरागविहितां सोढुं प्रणामक्रियां
हस्तन्यासमिवोद्वहन्ति न गजस्यैरण्डवृक्षाड·कुराः।। ४१।।

The God of Temptation (Kāma-dhātupati) then disappeared and reappeared shortly in the garb of Buddha as an actor with thirty-two signs of a great man from a forest. It was most pleasing to the eyes and looked like a brilliantly produced (coloured) painting, drawing on a cloth showing Buddha with a halo accompained by Śāradvatīputra (Sāriputta), Maudgalyāyana, Ānanda (behind), Mahāśramaṇas like Mahākaśyapa, Aniruddha, Subhūti, etc., together with scores of monks. The actual text is as follows:

मारश्च वनगहनमनुप्रविश्य बुद्धरूपं कृत्वा नट इव सुरुचिरनेपथ्य-
स्तस्माद्वनगहनादारब्धो निष्क्रमितुमि। वक्ष्यते हि —

ताथागतं वपुरथोत्तमलक्षणाढ्य -
मादर्शयन्नयनशान्तिकरं नराणम्।
प्रत्यग्रडरड·मिव चित्रपटं महार्ह -
मुद्घाटयन् वनमसौ तदलंचकार।। ४३।।

अथ व्योमप्रभामण्डलमण्डितमसेचनककदर्शनं भगवतो रुपमभिनिर्माय दक्षिणे पार्श्वे स्थविरशारद्वतीपुत्रं वामपार्श्वे स्थविरमहामौद्गल्यायनं पृष्ठतश्चायुष्मन्तमानन्दं बुद्धपात्रव्यग्रहस्तं स्थविरमहाकाष्यपानिरुद्धसुभूतिप्रभृतीनां च महाश्रावकाणां रुपाण्यभिनिर्माय अर्धत्रयोदशभिर्भिक्षुशतैरर्धचन्द्रेणानुपरिवृतं बुद्धवेषमादर्शयित्वा मारः स्थविरोपगुप्तस्यन्तिकमाजगाम।

Seeing this pleasant spectacle, Upagupta was thrilled and got up with folded hands to pay homage and then he also condemned the impermanent nature of things which destroys the *rūpa,* including even that of Buddha. The *Avadāna* beautifully describes the majestic form of Buddha bearing a golden lustre as seen by Upagupta which was full of grace and spotless beauty looking like a flower-garden, having the calm of the ocean and gait of a lion.

cf. 'स बुद्धावलम्बनया स्मृत्या तथाप्यासक्तमनाः संवृतो यथा बुद्धं भगवन्तमहं पश्यामीति व्यत्मुपागतः। स पद्यमुकुलप्रतिममत्रलिं कृत्वोवाच -- अहो रुपशोभा भगवतः। किं बहुना ?

'वक्रेणाभिभवत्ययं हि कमलं नीलोत्पलं चक्षुषा
कान्त्या पुष्पवनं धनं. प्रियतया चन्द्रं समाप्तद्युतिम्।
गाम्भीर्येण महोदधिं स्थिरतया मेरु रविं तेजसा
गत्या सिंहमवेक्षितेन वृषभं वर्णेन चामीकरम्।। ४५।।

Upagupta, feeling the presence of the Lord Buddha, forgot that it was an illusion and prostrated like a fallen trunk of a tree in front of the figure of Buddha. When Māra reminded him of his promise the monk said that he had paid homage to Buddha and not to Māra, although he knew that the Blessed One was no more. The monk, further, told that when people worship earthen images, they actually bow to the god, represented by the icons and not earthen form itself, and his action, therefore, was similar only to this kind of worship and that he detested (even) the thought of Māra and had, in fact, bowed only to Sugata oı Buddha (visible through body of Māra).

मृण्मयेषु प्रतिकृतिष्वमराणां यथा जनः।
मृतसंज्ञामनादृत्य नमत्यमरसंज्ञया।। ४६।।
तथाहं त्वामिहोद्वीक्ष्य लोकनाथवपुर्धरम्।
मारसंज्ञामनादृत्य नतः सुगतसंज्ञया।। ५०।।

Māra then came in his actual form and invited people to listen to Upagupta's discourse.

It is necessary to assess the contents of the *Avadāna* in the light of known facts of history. During the third century B.C., Upagupta might have been a historical personality who might have interpreted the Law of Buddha in one or the other way; but the story of subjugation of Māra by Upagupta appears to have been an addition made deliberately by the followers of Sarvāstivāda Sect to introduce and justify the worship of Buddha's representation in anthropomorphic form. This is evident from Upagupta's reference to the prevailing worship of earthen images of various deities. The need of such an action was most probably felt at Mathura by Sarvāstivādins. Most probably Aśvaghosha, the earliest Buddhist poet in Sanskrit, was the author of *Aśokāvadāna* for it tallies to a great extent with the contents of Aśvagosha's *Sutrālaṅkāra* even in the translated form. Therefore, Aśvaghosha, who seems to be leader of such a movement, may have given to the events connected with the life of Upagupta a mythological colour in a poetical language on account of the mounting pressure of Bhakti movement in Mathura and elsewhere as the *Avadāna* clearly mentions that even with slightest Bhakti it is possible to attain *nirvāna.*

(न्यायेनानेन भक्तिस्तव हृदिजनिता तेनाग्रमतिना
स्वल्पापि क्षत्र भक्तिर्भवति मतिमतां निर्वाणफलदा...
.... ।।३६।।)

In the great Buddhist Council held under the patronage of Kanishka (I) at Kuṇḍala-Vana Mahāvihāra, with which Aśvagosha was also associated as its Vice-President, perhaps, approved the idea to introduce the worship of the representation of Buddha in human form.

A similar tradition about Buddha figure painted on the basis of his shadow on a cloth at the instance of Bimbisāra during Master's life time in *Rudrāyaṇāvadāna* (part of *Divyāvadāna)* also confirms the existence of a movement to propagate the worship of Buddha's sculpture in human form.

It is due to this reason that early anthropomorphic depictions of Buddha are available both in Mathura and Gandhāra at the same time. The spread of this movement to important Buddhist centres in Madyadeśa is further attested to by records of monk Bala and nun Buddhamitrā inscribed around the early years of Kanishka (I)'s reign at Sarnath, Kauśāmbī and Śrāvastī which refer to the installation of Bodhisattva images (Sircar 1965: 135-37; 144-45), although similar to the representations of Buddha. The only exception in this regard is the inscribed but undated Buddha image from Anyor (Mathura) which is stylistically ascribed to the period of Kanishka I.

What we intend to emphasize is that through the episodes like the one of Upagupta and Māra presented in the *Aśokāvadāna,* the Buddhists of the Sarvāstivāda school attempted to project the importance of Buddha's *Rūpakāya* to incorporate the ideals of Bhakti in the concept which had already become an integral part of Buddhism by Kushan times. In this episode, even the Māra, the enemy of Buddha in a way is utilized for a noble cause generating an intense devotion to the Blessed One. Thus, the narration of such stories amongst the public by Dharma-Bhāṇakas (narrators of Dharma) and efforts made by monks like Bala in setting-up the Buddha images under the name of Bodhisattva may have convinced to a large extent orthodox Buddhist of Ganga-Yamuna region to accept Buddha's representation in human form as an object of worship to achieve heaven, material well-being, supreme knowledge and *nirvāṇa.*

REFERENCES

Dutta, Nalinaksha. 1953. *Saddharmapuṇḍarikasūtram.* Revised with N.D. Mironov's readings from Central Asian Mss. Calcutta.

Joshi, M.C. 1989. Aspects of Mauryan and Early Post-Mauryan Art in *Journal of the Indian Society of Oriental Art.* New Series. Calcutta. XVI, XVII.

Sharma, R.C. 1984. *Buddhist Art of Mathura. Delhi.*

Sircar, D.C. 1965. *Select Inscriptions.* 2nd edition. Calcutta.

Vaidya, P.L. (ed.). 1959. Divyāvadānam. Mithila. Also Sujit Kumar Mukhopadhyaya (ed., annotated and partly translated). *Aśokāvadāna.* New Delhi.

The Role of Computer in Archaeology

APARNA SENGUPTA*

Any study whose concepts are rooted in facts obtained from biosphere and which requires specialized techniques for a thorough examination and investigation of these facts, must justifiably belong to the class of science. Archaeology, says Graham Brade-Birks, is the science of man's past. According to Jason Smith, archaeology today has become as much an interdisciplinary science as it is a science unto itself. On the other hand, in the opinion of Glyn Daniel, archaeology cannot rightly be called a science nor a social science either. It is merely a technique for factual analysis of materials unearthed of man's past and serves as substruction for reconstruction of history. If the consensus is to treat archaeology as a branch of science, then it is a moot point that no aspect of science can be studied as an isolated subject. And to be able to grasp the true nature of a scientific subject the student must have some understanding of allied subjects which assist in enriching his knowledge about that particular area of science. Such subjects are denoted by the term 'inter-disciplines'. To be more precise, the study of interdisciplinary subjects provide the necessary background for a complete understanding of any branch of learning, whether it be arts, sciences or humanities. The point here is to what extent can an interdisciplinary science aid in the interpretation of archaeological studies and simplify its processing. A tool that achieves this objective (and much more besides) is the computer, an electronic wizard that solves several issues besides those that are addressed to it.

Before expanding on the several tasks that a computer can perform in the area of archaeology, it is of import to find out what precisely is the intended goal of an archaeologist.

Archaeologists excavate the material remains of past cultures and, by studying the evidence gathered by this exercise, they attempt to recreate the history of man from his earliest past, and so determine the nature of cultural systems at different times and places. In recent years archaeologists have realized the value of working together with scholars from other scientific disciplines such as geology, paleontology, climatology and so on. This enables the archaeologist to get a fuller picture of the culture he is trying to understand.

An important aspect of archaeological operations is the classification of materials obtained from the excavation of places, termed 'sites'. Based on such classifications, theories are formulated about how man lived in the past. One of the essential characteristics of such classification is the grouping of the material remains of various types such as classes, kinds, modes, schools, cultural periods, regions, etc. This is important in order to impart coherence to the data that are often multifarious in content, and which must be organized according to a pattern to enable the archaeologist to draw conclusions from. There are many ways in which this information can best be recorded, stored and dessiminated. One method is to break up this data into smaller groups, each possessing attributes common to all members of that group. Most archaeological constructs are founded on the study of such groups. It is here that the computer has an important role to play. Computer-oriented research in archaeology is a recent development and its popularity is gaining ground rapidly. This is because the computer opens up new areas of studies which the student of archaeology had hitherto thought unattainable. The computer's memory or storage bank constitutes an infinitely more reliable repository than the human memory both in respect of accuracy and the amount of information it can store. This is an immense advantage considering the corpus of often unrelated data that an archaeologist has to sift and collate for arriving at logical conclusions.

* C/o Editor, *Puratattva*, Archaeological Survey of India, Janpath, New Delhi.

The principal purpose of a computer in any situation is to record, store, retrieve and process large quantities of information. In essence, the computer's role consists in organizing any data and making sense out of it. Information retrieved during the course of excavations form a kind of jigsaw puzzle that needs to be uncoiled and a pattern produced of the finds obtained. For instance, when an item of artifact has to be analysed or a site has to be dated, it is necessary to relate the information to that obtained from other sites and other similar artifacts. For instance, previously artifacts were studied as isolated subjects; they were classified according to types and were sought to be described in relation to the regions and other associated assemblages. Now there is a swing towards new methods and approaches and a reassessment of the goals that need to be achieved. With the advancements in related fields archaeologists have recognized the need to broaden their vision and utilize the services of savants from all these fields to bring forth an integrated view of cultures as functional wholes rather than as mere sequences of artifacts, traits or assemblages.

More than the data however, the archaeologist's involvement in collecting and the interpretative techniques he applies are of primary importance. Admittedly, the computer lightens his work immensely. It prepares lists of various kinds of sites, of artifacts, of bibliographical sources with great speed and accomplishes correlations between the variety of finds unearthed.

But the computer has no brain and therefore cannot think. Therefore, in order to give satisfactory results the information entered must be consistent and questions addressed to it must be logical; only then can logical and correct results be obtained from it. Further, the computer cannot detect errors in logic, it can only check errors in syntax. Hence, if the information is entered wrongly the result will also be meaningless. There must also be no confusion regarding the data fed in. Unlike manual recording, computerization requires that the data be entered in a precise manner. Thus, for instance, if entries are being made, from all sites, of a particular type of pottery, each time the type occurs it must be put in the exact sequence (NBPW). Supposing the pottery type to be Northern Black Polished Ware, with the first letter of all the words in capital, it must be so each time. When a retrieval of this kind of pottery is required, the question will be put in a manner so that this particular information is accessed. If we enter this same detail differently at different times, there must be as many questions addressed to the computer. This quite defeats the purpose of computerization which is to hasten sorting and listing of multiple data types.

Most archaeological finds have a series of attributes, each of which may have similarity with like finds from another site. These attributes have to be sorted and listed for comparative searches at a future date. Attempted manually the listing would require describing the items in their full forms. The task can be both tedious and time consuming. Computerization of the same information consists in tabulating them in a specialized and analytical language or codes. The codes may be presented in any manner, as a combination of letters, digits or assorted form. The information thus entered comprises what is called a file of data. In the computer's memory each kind of information is stored in a particular way. Thus similar features of various items get clubbed together and when a list of a particular feature of all the items is required, a question is addressed to the machine whereby such a list is made available in a split second. This action, called selective retrieval, saves many hours of search through all the sites that would otherwise become inevitable. Let us take a single example. For instance, in the case of artifacts these attributes are generally size, raw material, type, decoration, etc. But how an item is described has a great bearing on the conclusions that can be drawn from its attributes. Two people might stress two different aspects of the same item and so give rise to two entirely different theories. Theories are built on those aspects that are prominent, and two individuals may give prominence to divergent aspects of an item leading to two different conclusions. For example two people given a hoard of the same punch-marked coins might give prominence to two different aspects of the coins - one to the location of their find and the other to the legends on them - depending on what inference each is trying to make of these coins. With a computer there is scarcely a chance for confusion as it will merely examine the attributes and slot them in their appropriate places. But as stated earlier, the manner of putting in the data must be consistent for foolproof inferences to be made.

What has been noted above refers to simple recording, storing and retrieval of data. More often the computer achieves tasks of a complex nature. For, archaeological information needs to be processed and statistical analyses have to be made to form ideas of cultural patterns at different points of time. To achieve this single objective, the archaeologist would have to take recourse to multiple activities for a clear cut presentation of several types of details from hundreds of sites, such as making diverse indexes of site attributes, photographs, charting maps of sites and so on. In the process, sometimes important details may very easily escape the memory of the person jotting them. The problems do not end here. After recording details, the next step is to sort the voluminous data for obtaining a clear picture of each detail. It is obvious that if the process has to be repeated for numerous sites, the exercise becomes sheer drudgery, while the results obtained are likely to be inaccurate as well as incomplete at places. The potential of a computer in such a situation can be easily realized.

In applying the computer for any job it is necessary to write what is called a program. The efficiency and effective use of the computer depends upon the quality of the programs used - both in terms of design and instructions. A computer program is a series of statements written in a particular sequence for producing exactly the kind of result that one wants from the file of information stored inside it. A program drawn out to meet the needs of a particular problem is called a software or package. There is as yet no special package in the market for archaeological data in the sense of a representative software that would cater to any and every kind of archaeological problem, as also organize the great variety of items obtained. Each problem is unique and the program written for it has to be so oriented that it answers all the possible questions that are put to it. But there does exist software in allied fields such as the natural and social sciences that can be used in archaeology for statistical and analytical work. But archaeological data also comprises details for which quantitative analyses are not appropriate. These deal with objects of art such as monuments, sculptures and even inscriptions. Yet here too the computer can serve a useful purpose in preparing an array of attributes that can ultimately be sorted in the same manner as artifacts and conclusions arrived at that help interpretations.

I will now discuss certain areas where the computer is being used in making a variety of deductions.

An important operation which plays a significant role in the archaeologist's task of tracking man's past is the decipherment of ancient writings. While advances in this area had already been made using other scientific techniques, much before the computer's ability was recognised, the computer's entry into the field made it possible for large-scale employment of statistical methods.

The computer was applied cautiously, on an experimental basis, at the USSR Academy of Sciences, where it was used to interpret the Maya hieroglyphic texts. However, Maya writing had been deciphered earlier by, what in computer jargon is called, 'manual' methods. The purpose of using the computer for obtaining results that were already in evidence, was to verify the machine's ability to solve such complex problems. The manual results were, therefore, used as control.

In the computation of undeciphered scripts, the first requisite is the preparation of a concordance of sign-occurrences and tabulation of frequencies of signs and symbols occurring in the text.

In the experiment carried out at the Academy of Sciences, the goal was to establish a relationship between the words of the lexicon and the texts, and of determining the meaning of the hieroglyphs. A series of operations were undertaken. The frequency of the syllables were, compared with the frequencies of the symbols in the text, and lists were made of words matching with the meanings. For hieroglyph as related to drawings, a list of synonyms were prepared and the one that appeared most accurate was chosen.

As evident from the nature of the operations undertaken, the information compiled was enormous. The data, when processed, gave the same results as that shown by the manual methods. In other words, it yielded no new facts. While this might, at face value, be taken as a point unfavorable to the machine's ability, in actual truth, the results of the experiment confirm the view that computer technology can be employed successfully in analysing ancient scripts.

Nearer home, attempts were made to interpret the Indus Script. The method was developed at the Computer Center of the College of Engineering, Guindy, Madras, and the computer used was the IBM 1620 Model II Electronic Digital Computer. For typesetting of the script and printing of the texts and concordances, a more sophisticated computer had to be used. This was made available at the National Center for Software Development and Computing Technique (NCSDCT) at TIFR, Bombay.

The analysis was conducted in several stages. For the first stage of the work, that of preparing sign-concordance, distribution charts were drawn tabulating the frequencies of sitewise and typewise occurrences of inscribed objects and positional frequency of signs and sign-combinations. For the statistical part of the analysis, inscriptions on seals, sealings, graffiti, and other miscellaneous objects such as bronze weapons, dice, copper tablets, etc., were compiled as lines of text.

Each line of a data had three constituents - a sequence number, a background data consisting of the various factors relevant to the data, namely, the site, the location of the object within the site, the type of the object, associated 'field symbols' found on the object (eg. 'Unicorn', 'Humped Bull'), the number of inscribed sides, the number of inscribed lines, and the length and direction of each line-the latter has generally been found earlier to run from right to left.

The sign were coded as a series of 3-digit numbers, lines of text being arranged in the sequence of these numbers. Since the script is not a deciphered one, it was immaterial what the original direction of writing was. Therefore, in the coded text the lines run from left to right. One line of text comprises a 6-digit sequences number, 14-digit background data and a 45-digit text (Col. 21-80.) Input cards were first sorted according to a decided pattern, from these then output cards were prepared, whence the signs were rearranged in a specific order with reference to their sequence numbers. (In general, all sorting was done in an ascending order of numerical sequence).

In order to read the data, the different sign were sorted repeatedly, and tables prepared of signs immediately preceding and succeeding each sign, both in a numerical sequence.

The script did contain not only single signs, but paired as well as combinations of pairs. All these were treated in a similar manner as with the individual signs. Tables were also prepared of the positional frequencies of signs which might give a clue to the probable nature of the language.

Although the exact nature of the text could not be deduced immediately from the initial experiments, it provided valuable guidelines for future tests to be carried out along these lines.

The purpose of the experiment with the Indus Script was to find out the frequencies of the various signs embedded in the text. The results of the experiment showed that only a handful of signs, out of nearly 400, occurred most frequently, leading to the conclusion that they probably formed the core of the script. Figures 1-4 illustrate some of the operations carried out on this script and a sample output of the concordance and text.

An area where the computer has made great strides is in graphics. Computer graphics means presenting a pictorial output of information basically statistical or mathematical in content. The illustration may be in the form of a map, a picture or a graph.

As in an ordinary graph, the data is plotted along the X-Y coordinates. For this a mechanical drawing device, called a plotter, is used to describe the picture that has to be displayed. Plotters are of two main types, the drum plotter, in which the pen moves only on one axis and the paper has to be rotated for the other axis; the second is the flatbed plotter which moves on both axes. The display obtained by a plotter can be altered as desired - for making additions, deletions, or rotated to give a 3-dimentional effect.

There are several applications of graphics in archaeology, such as in drawing of artifact shapes and several kinds of distribution charts like site distribution, map-base illustration, contour maps and so on. Let us take a single example, that of artifact shapes. Graphics can greatly assist in forming an idea of successive patternings of behaviour that were responsible for giving a particular shaped rim to a vessel, and show how this rim changed with changes in the different cultural periods. The use of graphics allows manipulating this data : in various ways, viz., enlarging or contracting the picture or obtaining simultaneous display of different kinds of rims for comparison. In the same way, artifact distribution within a particular site can be studied by plotting the attributes of an artefact like raw material, technique and morphological characteristics. Discrete groups of the same artifact are thus formed based on these attributes. Several conclusions can be drawn from this. For instance, the raw material might belong to one period, while the technique may belong to another, which would mean that there was an overlapping of two cultural periods. In other words, the particular type of artifact probably comes from a transitory period when there was not much change in the raw material which, perhaps, came from a single source. Such an experiment was carried out by the IBM in 1971. They conducted a project to record vessel shape and decoration of about 2000 Egyptian vessels in the Metropolitan Museum of Art in New York.

There are a great number of prepared package for conducting computer-graphics surveys, but these have to be tested first as graphics require precision.

The ability of a computerized input to adjust to changes in information is one of its great advantages. Whereas a book or article is static, a computer data-base can be continuously expanded to incorporate new information as and when they become available. Newly discovered artifacts can be slotted into their appropriate places.

Finally, a word of caution seems appropriate. If the results obtained from a computer are accepted uncritically it would defeat the objective of the archaeologist. For, the results obtained from a computer are only as good as the evidence upon which they are based. Their great advantage, apart from saving time, is to enable the archaeologists to arrive at quicker and surer hypotheses that would otherwise depend largely on intuition. Above all, a computer analysis can take a lot of confusing details into account and weigh them consistently without the pre-conceived notions of any archaeologist. But, the archaeologist must remain the final judge of the findings and their organization into the computer must be checked often for the results produced to be accurate and meaningful.

REFERENCES

Antiquity. Volume 63. Number 238. March 1989.

Antiquity. Volume 63. Number 239. June 1989.

Advances in Archaeology. Volume 5. New York. 1982.

Agrawal, D.P. and Ghosh A. 1973 *Radiocarbon and Indian Archaeology*. TIFR. Bombay.

Brade-Birks, S. Graham. 1957. *Archaeology*. Teach yourself Books. London.

Ceram, C.W. 1966. *The world of Archaeology*. London.

Deetz, James. 1967. *Invitation to archaeology*. American Museum Science Books. New York.

Greene, Kevin. 1983. *Archaeology - An introduction*. New Jersey.

Hole, Frank and Robert F. Heizer 1973. *Prehistoric Archaeology-A brief introduction*. U.S.A.

Krishna Rao, M.V.N. 1982. Indus script deciphered. New Delhi.

Mahadevan, I. 1977. *The Indus Script*. ASI. Memoir No. 77. New Delhi.

Srivastava, K.M. 1982. *New Era of Indian Archaeology*. New Delhi.

TABLE OF DISTRIBUTION OF INSCRIBED OBJECTS ACCORDING TO SITE AND TYPE

FREQUENCY RANGE	NO. OF SIGNS	TOTAL SIGN OCCURRENCES	PER CENT (OF TOTAL OCCURRENCES)
1000 or more	1	1395	10.43
999-500	1	649	4.85
499-100	31	6344	47.44
99-50	34	2381	17.81
49-10	86	1833	13.71
9-2	152	658	4.92
Only once	112	112	0.84
Total	417	13372	100.00

SITES	OBJECT TYPES*								TOTAL
	1	2	3	4	5	6	7	8	
Mohenjodaro	1232	119		13	135	5	28	8	1540
Harappa	350	288	272	64		3	1	7	985
Chanhudaro	58	3		4		1			66
Lothal	89	75		1					165
Kalibangan	56	21		20		2			99
Other sites	13	4		17					34
West Asian Finds	16	1							17
TOTAL	1814	511	272	119	135	11	29	15	2906

Fig. 1A -

*Note : The type codes represent: (1) seals, (2) sealings, (3) miniature stone, terracotta or faience tablets, (4) pottery graffiti, (5) copper tablets, (6) bronze implements, (7) ivory or bone rods and (9) miscellaneous inscribed objects.

POSITION	NO. OF SIGNS	TOTAL FREQUENCY
Solus	88	190
Initial	290	3010
Medial	286	7196
Final	173	2976
Total	417*	13372

* A sign can occur in more than one position.

Fig. 1B - TABLE OF POSITIONAL DISTRIBUTION OF SIGNS WITH RESPECT TO LINES OF TEXT

A sing can occur in four possible positions, viz. solus (one sign constituting the whole line), initial, medial or final.

1-4	5	6	7-8	9	10
2405	1	1	01	0	1
		2	00	1	2
				2	1
		3	00	0	1
		4	00	0	1
		5	00	0	3
		6	00	0	9

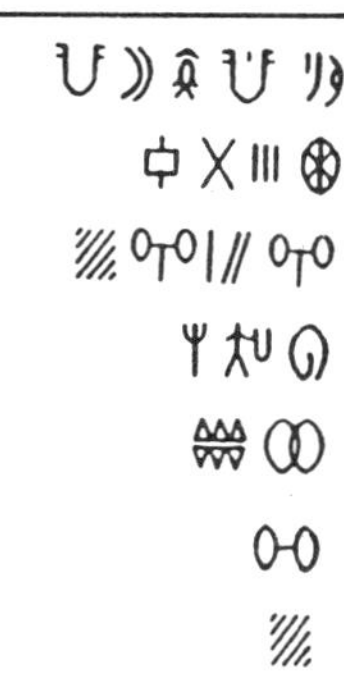

Explanations:

COL. NO.	DESCRIPTION	CODE	KEY
1-4	Text number	2405	FEM 405*
5	Type	1	Seal
6	Side number	1-6	Sides 1 to 6
7-8	Field symbol	01	Unicorn (on side 1)
		00	Nil (on other sides)
9	Line number	0	Only line (on sides 1, 3-6)
		1	First line (on side 2)
		2	Second line (on side 2)
10	Direction of writing	1	Right to left
		2	Left to right
		3	Only sign in the line
		9	Doubtful

Note: The symbol  indicates illegible or lost passages with one or more signs. The line of text on the sixth side is wholly illegible, but included as other lines of the same text are legible.

* FEM 405: E.J.H. Mackay, Further Excavations at Mohenjodaro, Delhi.

Fig. 2: A specimen passage from the Text (2405)

Sometimes seals are found inscribed not only on one or both the flat faces but also on the edges (e.g. 2405). Each such inscribed surface is regarded as a 'side' of the inscribed object in question.

MOHENJODARO

1066	100101	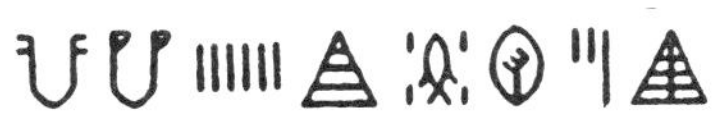
1067	100101	
1068	100101	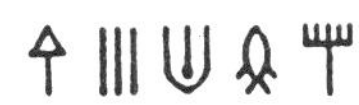
1069	100101	
1070	100101	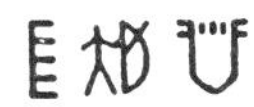
1071	100101	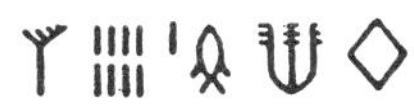
1072	100101	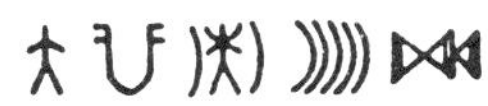
1073	100109	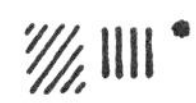
1074	100101	
1075	100101	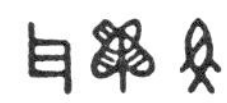
1076	100101	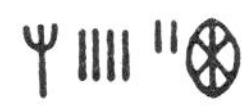
1077	100101	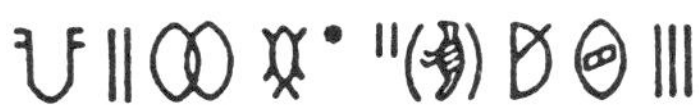
1078	100101	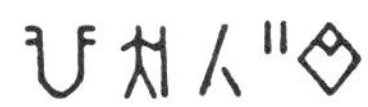
1079	100101	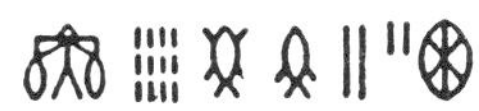
1080	100101	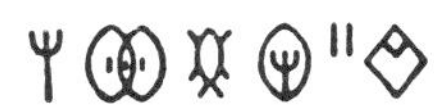
1081	100101	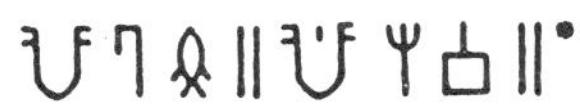
1082	100101	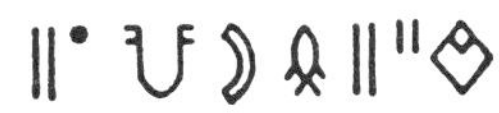
1083	100101	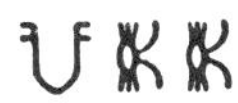
1084	100101	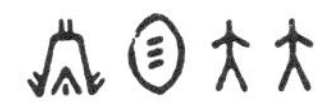
1085	100101	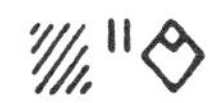
1086	100101	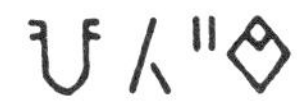

1087	100101	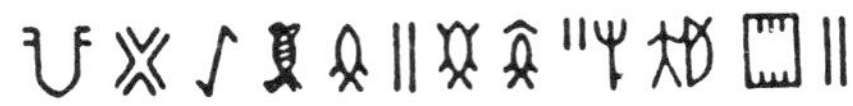
1088	100101	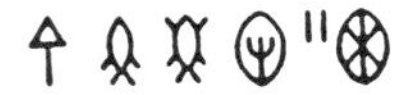
1089	100101	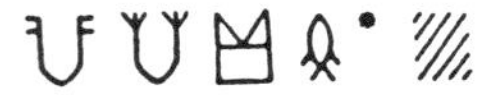
1090	100101	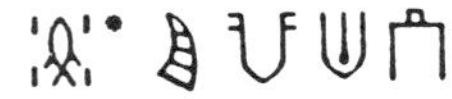
1091	100101	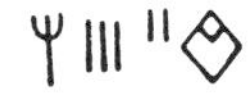
1092	100101	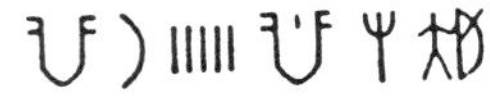
1093	100113	
	25	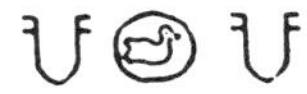
	31	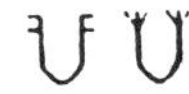
1094	100101	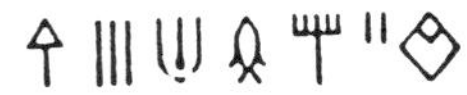
1095	100101	
1096	100101	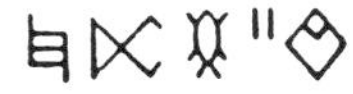

CONCORDANCE

4712	00	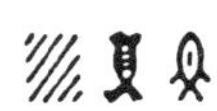
3307	00	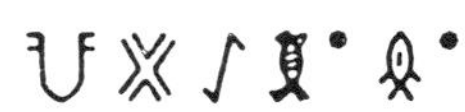
1370	00	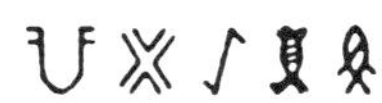
4683	10	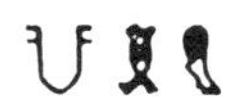
	20	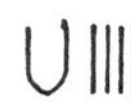
4500	10	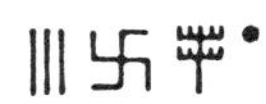
	20	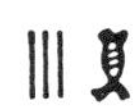
4482	10	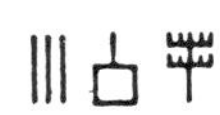
	20	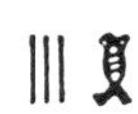
4486	10	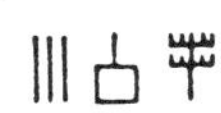
	20	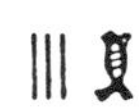
1309	00	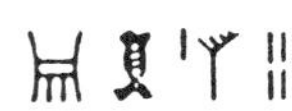

4118	00
2424	00
4375	10
	20
2229	10
	20
2109	00
8006	00
4717	10
	20
4595	10
	20
4348	10
	20
9701	10
	20
	30
2690	01
	02
1012	01
	02

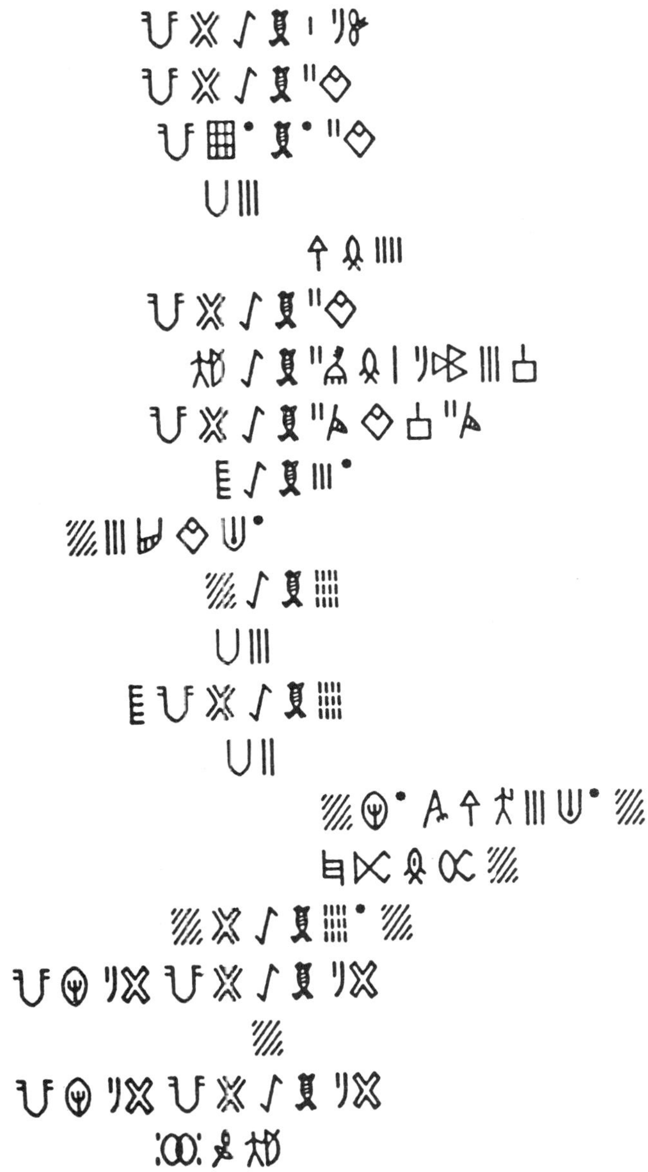

A SPECIMEN OF CODED LINES OF TEXT (INPUT DATA)

1-6	7-8	9-11	12	13	14-16	17-18	19-20	21-80		
100102	23	-03	1	3	501	05	04	000	125	131
100101	23	-03	1	1	501	01	01	346	008	147

Explanation:

Col. No.	Data	Code	Key
1	Site	1	Mohenjodaro (Marshall)
2-4	Object Number	001	Marshall (1931) Seal No. 1
5	Side number	0	Only side
6	Line Number	1,2	Lines 1 & 2
7-8	Location	23	Lower city - HR area
9-11	Level	-03	3 below surface
14-16	Field Symbol	501	Animal (Unicorn?) facing right (as on impression)
17-18	Number of positions in the line		05, 01 5 positions (one position in the 2nd line)
19-20	Length of line	04	4 signs (extant) in one line 1 sign in line 2
21-80	Coded text	000	Broken portion of line 1

The Legacy of Indus Civilization in North India

K.N. DIKSHIT*

Since the discovery of the Indus Civilization in the 1920s which opened a new chapter of India's past and put back its antiquity to the 3rd millennium B.C., there has been speculation on the extent to which this civilization has influenced the Indian culture materially and spiritually or the second urbanization in Ganga valley could be a survival or revival of Indus urbanism.

The excavations at Harappa, Mohenjodaro, Chanhudaro, Lothal, Surkotada, Kalibangan and Banawali revealed the salient features of this civilization in the form of a systematic layout of cities, well regulated drainage system and bathrooms, use of standard sized burnt-bricks, steatite seals depicting the animal kingdom, with pictographic or ideographic script, animal and human terracotta figurines, terracotta cakes, chert blades and weights and bronze objects. The Harappan pottery is characterized by a well burnt black painted red ware with distinctive shapes like dish-on-stand, cylindrical vase, perforated jar, goblet, storage jar etc. The general motifs on the pottery are intersecting circles, leaf and fish-scale patterns and human and animal figurines.

We know for certain that the end of Indus civilization was not abrupt and final as thought earlier, but it rolled down and passed on earlier aspects to a subsequent culture which could be called 'Sub-Indus Cultures'. The areas like Gujarat and north India produced material to highlight continuity and change specially in reconstructing the post Indus phase. Even in nuclear area, new look at Jhukar, Jhangar and Cemetery H cultures has given a new idea of Indus survival (Mughal 1984: 499-503, Dani 1981: 10). The Indus legacy, if any, has to be understood in the perspective of what follows during the post Indus phase down to the beginning of historical period.

The Mature Indus phase degenerated into a well defined Late phase which was reflective of changes (Dales 1966: 98). To be precise this phase marked the end of writing, use of weights and measures, construction of monumental buildings and idea of town-planning but at the same time it followed the cultural continuity of Mature Harappan and its associated miscellany. The transformation or process of degeneration of Harappa culture into poor sub-Indus cultures in Gujarat and Saurashtra is an accepted phenomenon but in Jammu and Kashmir, Haryana, Punjab and western Uttar Pradesh this picture has emerged only in the last two three decades (Dikshit 1979: 123-133). This phase is identified with the end of city life and has been placed at the moment somewhere in a flexible time bracket between 1800 B.C. and 1200 B.C.

Against this background the legacy of the Indus civilization in the field of material or immaterial things handed down from predecessors has been examined. The question comes to mind that what happened to the lingering elements of this civilization after its collapse and in what way did Indus religion and mythology influence the religious ideas and mythology of later Indian culture. It was argued that many later-day Hindu religio-ritualistic practices and

* Archaeological Survey of India, Janpath, New Delhi.

Paper read in the conference of South Asian Archaeology at Paris in 1989. I wish to acknowledge the useful suggestions of Prof. B.B. Lal and constructive criticism of my colleagues -- Dr. S.P. Gupta, J.P. Joshi and M.C. Joshi.

spiritual thoughts were derived from Indus civilization. However, there is a school of thought which believes that there was a complete break in tradition and no continuity of the lingering elements of the Indus civilization in the contemporary and succeeding chalcolithic cultures is seen. We need not agree with this view but at the same time we must examine the claim for how all the urban traits of this civilization ceased to exist simultaneously with the end of cities.

G.R. Sharma claimed from his excavations at Kausambi (District Allahabad) that the architecture of the fortifications and drain at Kausambi was borrowed from that of Indus civilization (Sharma 1960). The mud packed rempart revetted externally with baked bricks in the so called English bond in alternate courses of headers and stretchers, rectangular towers and underground passage built on corbelled arch are significant features of architecture at Kausambi. The defences show that in the first centuries of the first millennium B.C., Kausambi developed as a town fully equipped for its protection by the magnificient defences built on the Harappan pattern. Even the pottery obtained from the lowest levels of the defences and palace areas was connected with Harappan echo/or influence. This statement led us believe the continuity of Harappan tradition in mid Ganga valley where the very idea of town life was so far unknown.

This statement of Sharma was challenged by K.K. Sinha, A. Ghosh and also by B.B. Lal saying that as no burnt brick structure prior to the NBPW period was noticed in Ganga valley, these defences cannot be placed to such an early antiquity. So was the case with the pottery from defences which could really lay claims to be called Harappan.

Lal, while reviewing this problem in a Conference on Harappan Civilization, was of the view that even if the Kausambi fortifications and drains are for a while accepted to have been derived from their counterparts at Harappa and Mohenjodaro respectively, one would have still to answer: how is it that only these two isolated features reached Kausambi without the brick sizes about which the Harappans were so meticulous'. He also raised the issue of the absence of grid-patterned town-planning (Lal 1982: 335-338). We may not emphasize the Harappan brick-sizes because along with the standard size, a few unconventional brick sizes also continued as one can see in the excavations of the Late Harappan sites - Hulas, Alamgirpur, Sanghol and a few others in north India. Even on Late Harappan sites the grid patterned town planning was a closed issue, except that the houses were built on a raised mud platform - a concept Harappans never left even in their movement to east or south-east from nuclear region.

However, one cannot discuss Indus legacy without referring the work of A. Ghosh. He has made a critical analysis about the survival or revival of the Indus urbanism. To quote 'Harappan urbanism could not have been remotely produced or inspired the historical urbanism, for the simple reason that there is no perceptible link between the Harappa and later Indian cultures. There are wide gaps, either temporal or spatial or both, for any infiltration to have possibly taken place. So far as it can be discerned at present, the Indian style could not have taken its origin before the spread of Sanskritization, when only the Great Tradition and the Little Tradition of Indian culture met, mixed with and interacted upon each other' (Ghosh 1973: 85). Thapar, while examining the distinctive traits of the Indus civilization and the salient features of the cultural equipment of other contemporary and succeeding chalocolithic cultures also does not see any continuity from the Indus civilization (Thapar 1976: 1-4). Possehl, who discussed the post-urban Harappan phase is also of the view that the so called 'Second Urbanization' of north India is not to be seen as a process involving the institutions of the Harappan urban phase because it lies well outside this socio-cultural environment (Possehl and Raval 1989: 19).

Allchins on the other hand are of the opinion that Indus religion and mythology have greatly contributed to the religious ideas and mythology of later Indian culture even long after the first cities had disappeared (Allchins 1982). However, to substantiate this statement by concrete examples is difficult. The Northern Nuclear Region (Punjab, Haryana and Indo-Gangetic divide) · forming a continuous geographical zone according to Allchins provide a continuing interaction between the local cultural style and that of Indus region. However, on examination it was noticed that even this process appears to have remained confined within the period of decline of this civilization and not beyond.

To quote Gupta 'When an urban culture declines with external political interference, as was the case with the Harappans, the cultural items which are prone to persist include basic crafts relating to stone, bone and clay as well as the knowledge of agriculture and animal husbandry. It may also include, in some areas at least crafts like metallurgy and glazing (faience). But the most important item which we may not always be in a position to prove archaeologically save indirectly, is the preservation of oral traditions' (Gupta 1982: 56). However, with the arrival of Aryans on Indian scene to isolate oral traditions is difficult.

To understand the Indus legacy one has to go through with its dispersal. The cultural gamut of the nuclear region - the Indus Ghaggar Divide - when compared internally revealed regional variations conforming to devolutionary tendencies specially in the peripheral region of north India. A very large number of sites what are now loosely termed as 'Late Harappan' have been discovered. These sites which formed the disrupted terminal phases of the culture lost their status as Harappan. They no doubt yielded distinctive Harappan pottery, antiquities and remnants of some architectural forms but no town planning nor any economic and cultural nucleus. The Indus script also disappeared.

A survey of some of the excavated sites and other exploratory field data in north India, namely, Manda in Jammu and Kashmir; Kotla Nihang Khan, Ropar, Chandigarh, Bara, Dher Majra, Sanghol, Katpalon, Nagar and Dadheri in Punjab; Mitathal, Banawali, Balu, Mirzapur, Daulatpur and Bhagwanpura in Haryana and Alamgirpur, Bargaon and Hulas in Uttar Pradesh have provided sufficient material for understanding the settlement pattern and other social and cultural aspects including the chronological framework of the Harappan vis-a-vis Late Harappan cultures. To examine the legacy issue, only such features of the newly excavated sites, as are relevant to the issue, are being mentioned here:

Manda, District Akhnoor (Jammu and Kashmir)

Manda is located on the right bank of the river Chenab. The sub period IA is identified with Harappans living in circular or semi-circular huts, mud walled houses and houses of baked brick or jelly whereas sub period IB is associated with Harappan red ware and grey ware of Painted Grey Ware assemblage.

Dadheri, District Ludhiana (Punjab)

The excavations at Dadheri reveled a three fold sequence of cultures. The sub-period IA is represented by Late Harappan Culture closely followed by sub-period IB having Late Harappan and Painted Grey Ware together.

Nagar and Katpalon, District Jullundhur (Punjab)

The lowest Period I of both these sites corresponds to sub-period IB of Dadheri.

Bhagwanpura, District Kurukshetra (Haryana)

It revealed a two fold sequence of cultures. In sub-period IA, Late Harappans occupied this place, whereas in sub-period IB arrival of PGW users was noticed in Late Harappan Culture - complex.

Alamgirpur, District Meerut (U.P.)

The period I has typical Harappan pottery with cloth impressions on a trough. Two groups of kiln-burnt bricks and a short incised inscription consisting of two characters were found. After a break, the site was reoccupied by PGW users.

Hulas, District Saharanpur (U.P.)

The period I yielded Harappan red ware, besides the associated non-Harappan red and thick grey wares. The complex is marked by the absence of beakers and perforated jars and steatite beads and absence of any form of structures except solid mud platform and mud walled houses and huts. It has a terracotta sealing with three Harappan characters.

Ambkheri and Bahadarabad, District Saharanpur (U.P.)

These two sites which are on Ganga proper also form the part of degenerate Harappan gamut.

The devolution or gradual transformation of the Indus civilization from the Mature to the Late is very clear from Manda in north to Alamgirpur and Hulas in the east specially in pottery forms and minor works of art and craft (Dikshit 1984: 253-269). The Harappan Cemeteries like R-37 at Harappa, Lothal and Kalibangan are away from habitations. And so was the case with Ropar and Chandigarh. At Bhgwanpura, two skeletons lying in north-south orientation with heads towards the north, were found from the habitation area of sub-period IB. There are no funerary goods in the graves (Joshi and Madhu Bala 1982: 185-195).

The evidence from Bhagwanpura perhaps presents a transition from Bronze Age to Early Iron Age as noticed in Iran and Soviet Central Asia. However, there is no reflection of any Harappan tradition in successive cultures - the Painted Grey Ware or Northern Black Polished Ware.

The Survey revealed that the Indus civilization did not die a sudden death with the destruction of towns in the central Indus valley and Rajasthan, but its elements survived for many centuries even outside the Indus valley in Saurashtra and Gujarat, north Deccan, Malwa, Haryana, Punjab and western Uttar Pradesh (including Bahadarabad and Ambkheri). The date bracket of the sites from the Late Harappan to the inter-locking stage noticed with PGW comes up to the threshold of Iron Age. But the long gap between the end of Indus cities and the beginning of second urbanization i.e., the establishment of *Mahājanapadas* has provided a gap of over a thousand years, thereby suggesting no contact with the Harappan urban tradition.

The legacy of Indus civilization can be seen only in the conceptual continuity such as represented by symbols and motifs on Punch Marked Coins and like material including the representation of *Śiva-Paśupati*, *linga* and *mother goddess*. However, these are also far from convincingly proved (Ghosh 1973: 83). The Daimabad bronzes which are outside Harappan culture context perhaps owe some kind of technological survival to Harappans although it is difficult to substantiate.

From the foregoing survey, we may recall that much of the discussion centered on views for or against continuity but at the same time it could not also be proved that in what form the legacy of the Indus civilization continued and survived because in all probability this was also the time of the main movement of Indo-Aryans in India. The early Aryan society provided a firm base to the Hindu society, in which to separate Aryan and non-Aryan elements is not only difficult but impossible.

REFERENCES

Allchin, B. and Raymond. 1982. *The Rise of Civilization in India and Pakistan.* Cambridge. Cambridge University Press.

Dales, G.F. 1966. The Decline of Harappans. in *Scientific American* 214. 5. New York.

Dani, A.H. 1981. The Indus Civilization - New Perspectives in *Indus Civilization-New Perspectives.* Islamabad, Quaid-i-Azam University.

Dikshit, K.N. 1984. Late Harappa in Northern India. in *Frontiers of the Indus Civilization.* New Delhi. Books and Books.
1979. The Late Harappan Cultures in India, in *Essays in Indian Protohistory.* New Delhi. B.R. Publishing House.

Ghosh, A. 1973. *The City in Early Historical India.* Simla. Indian Institute of Advanced Study.

Gupta, S.P. 1982. The Late Harappan: A study in Cultural Dynamics. in *Harappan Civilization: A Contemporary Perspective.* New Delhi. Oxford and IBH.

Joshi, J.P. and Madhu Bala. 1982. Manda: A Harappan Site in Jammu and Kasnmır. in *Harappan Civilization: A contemporary Perspective.* New Delhi. Oxford and IBH.

Lal, B.B. 1982. West was West and East was East, but when and How Did the Twain Meet? The Role of Bhagwanpura as a Bridge between Certain Stages of the Indus and Ganges Civilizations. in *Harappan Civilization: A Contemporary Perspective.* New Delhi. Oxford and IBH.

Mughal, M.R. 1984. The Post-Harappan Phase in Bahawalpur District, Pakistan. in *Frontiers of Indus Civilization.* New Delhi. Books and Books.

Possehl, G.L. and M.H. Raval. 1989. *Harappan Civilization and Rojdi.* New Delhi. Oxford and IBH.

Sharma, G.R. 1960. *The Excavations at Kausambi (1957-59).* Allahabad. University of Allahabad.

Thapar, B.K. 1976. The End of the Indus Civilization and its Aftermath. in *Archaeological Congress and Seminar. 1972.* Kurukshetra. B.N. Chakravarti University. Kurukshetra.

Excavations at Karkabhat

A.K. SHARMA*

The megalithic site of Karkabhat, District Durg, (M.P.) is spread in an area of about 10 sq. km. encompassing the villages of Karhi Badar, Kanyawada, Muzhgahan, Sorar, Chirchari, Tengna, Nahanda and Karkabhat. The entire area is dotted by natural springs and minor nallahs. All the megaliths are located on the rocky outcrops and high areas. The rock shelters are dotted on the peaks of the boulder outcrops. Karkabhat (Lat. 20° 41′18", Long. 81° 19′ 7") is located 16 kms. from Balod on Balod-Dhamtari road. As per our assessment, there must have been nearly 3500 to 4000 megalithic burials in this area, major part of which have now been totally wiped out. At Karkhabat itself there are more than 800 such burials.

At Karkabhat, the megalithic memorials (pl. IX) of seven identified types, are densely concentrated near the two perennial springs. They are located in the high rock bench and thin soil cover area, in a monsoon fed lateritic zone, with the added advantage of having a large number of low natural rock shelters nearby. In the same area there are sprawling outcrops of trap and sandstone, where menhirs of different sizes and shapes are still lying in finished and unfinished condition. Apart from these geological and topographic considerations (1) location of megaliths at Karkabhat also appear to be influenced by the availability of iron, copper and gold. *Iron* ore deposits are confined to Dalli-Rajhara range of hills which are located nearly 20 kms. from Karkabhat. There are reserves in Dendi-Lohara also. Due to presence of several springs in the neighbourhood, iron ore is available in very pure form.

Encrustation of copper have been found near Chicholi and Warar-Band, not very far from the site.

Habitation area

So far evidence of habitational areas in megalithic sites have alluded investigations and nothing was known about their mode of living. At Karkhabat to the south and south-west of the burial area, there are a number of low rock shelters, each one sufficient enough to accommodate, during night and inclement weathers two persons. These rock shelters and caves also are spread in a large area, particularly to the south of the Karkabhat megaliths. Two or three rock shelters spotted at Bilai Dongri in the area of Nahanda village have occupational deposits of nearly 30 to 32 cms. which should reveal more details about the living pattern of megalithic people of this area.

Factory site

Between the rock shelters and the burial sites, is located the factory site for cutting out and shaping menhirs of different sizes and shapes. These menhirs have been found in different stages of preparation.

Burial site

The burial site is located north of the factory site and in between the two natural springs which were sources of constant supply of water.

On the basis of morphological features and layout seven types have been identified. They are three more than identified earlier (I.A.R. 1956-57) at a nearby site of Dhanora by M.G. Dikshit. The site has since been wiped out. The types identified are:

Type A. Stone cairn circle with loose packing, rising to a height of about 0.35 m. from the ground level.

Type B. Stone cairn circle with distinct cairn heap rising upto a height of 1 to 1.30m. from the ground level.

* Archaeological Survey of India, Prehistory Branch, Nagpur.

Type C. Stone cairn circle with a single menhir, small or big, in the centre of the circle and surrounded with heaped cairn packing.

Type D. Stone cairn circle with two menhirs erected side by side in the northern half of the circle and surrounded with heaped cairn packing.

Type E. Stone cairn circle with two menhirs, kept in the northern half and the other in the southern half of the circle, surrounded with heaped cairn packing.

Type F. Stone cairn circle with multiple menhirs of varying sizes kept in two rows, one in the northern half and the other row in the southern half of the circle. All the menhirs are surrounded with heaped cairn packing.

Type G. Stone cairn circle with cap-stone in the centre resting over a heap of stones. Cap stone oriented in north-south direction lengthwise.

In order to ascertain the significance of the above mentioned burial types one of each type has been taken up for excavation. During the course of excavation the following notable features have been observed.

1. All the circles and menhirs are oriented north-south, i.e. in case of circles, length is north-south whereas all menhirs are having their finished smooth surface facing north.
2. In most cases northern fringe of the cairn circle, upto nearly 1/3 of the circle, are lined with bigger size of boulders.
3 Presence of multiple stone circles of smaller size in the main cairn circle, with one or two stump like stones in the centre. In one case, these smaller circles belonging to different phases, have been noticed. From some of these smaller circles, pottery of thin grey ware and rough black and red ware have been recovered.
4 Presence of multiple stone circles within a bigger cairn circle and presence of multiple menhirs are indicative of family burial.

Architecture

Karkabhat megalithic people had an advanced knowledge of sepulchral architecture, involving cutting, shaping, transporting and erecting such huge menhirs as memorials. Even huge quantity of boulders were also transported and meticulously arranged around the menhirs. In case of multiple menhir memorials involving two or more than two menhirs care was taken to erect them at right place in the right direction and in case of multiple burials at equi-distance. Each cairn circle was lined with big boulders in the northern half and then at the bottom level a distinct circle of stones was made. This circle was enlarged with great precision with the induction of more menhirs in course of time. Even in case of single menhirs the successive layers of boulders were arranged in a pyramidal fashion slowly rising to the top. In each case right from the bottom the entire space around the menhirs/capstones, was filled with boulders arranged in circles with a central stone. Each stone of the circle formed another circle, in this way a number of circles were created filling the whole area. After the creation of first stage of circles the entire area was filled with yellow or red fine silt. Over the filling the process of making circle was again repeated. This was done till the filling reached the desired height. Thus number of circles from bottom to top in stages were created in a receding fashion. It is not clear whether this process was continued in a regular manner without break in course of few days months or was continued after breaks. The earlier possibility as per evidence appears to be more likely.

This method of raising the cairn height with circles and successive filling is a new feature observed. It is in one of these circles that the offerings were deposited.

Thus the megalithic people of Karkbhat adopted the circles and pyramidal form for creating cairn heights.

Sense of direction

Each menhir has been so erected that the finished surfaces face north and the unfinished south. These menhirs have been further subjected to putting them in east or west inclination. They have also been shaped in such a fashion that either they are conical pointing upwards or their top end is fashioned obliquely, the pointed end pointing either to the east or to the west. The angle of deviation from the magnetic north shows that they were deliberately so erected that they indicate direction and solar position. It is not necessary that these memorial menhirs were erected immediately after the death of the person. They might have been erected even after a lapse of time but that position indicates the time and period of year when the deceased left the world.

Shape of Menhirs

A. *Fish shaped*.- In this type one end is pointed whereas the other is bifurcated in the form of tail of a fish. In case of standing menhirs of this type bifurcated end is towards the top whereas in case of cap stones it is towards north.

B. *Obliquely pointed.*- Top of menhir is obliquely pointed with the pointed end towards east or west.

C. *Conical.*- The top of menhir is conical and erected in such a way that the magnetic line passes through the pointed end of the menhir.

Cultural equipment

Only few fragments of red ware were recovered from some of the excavated megaliths. The pottery is wheel made seemingly on a slow wheel and fired at a comparatively low temperature. Common shapes are bowls, dishes and lids. The ware shows a dull terracotta red surface with a pale drab slip. The core is generally unoxidized. Other distinctive element was the use of iron, copper, gold and silver.

The offerings recovered from the excavated megaliths are mostly iron objects, copper bangles and rings, gold rings, a silver ring and stone bead.

Iron objects

In all 13 iron objects were recovered.

Speardheads & Daggers	- 6
Arrow heads	- 4
Spikes	- 2
Agriculture implement	- 1

In the collection there are hardly any agricultural implements except one, which is probably a hoe, similar to one found at Ramapuram (pl. X). This indicates that the megalithic people of the area around Karkabhat did not practise agriculture on a settled scale but led a pastoral life. Rest of the iron objects are instruments of defence and attack (pl. XI).

Copper objects

Copper objects recovered are mostly in the form of rings and bangles of different sizes. They are all solid. The rings and bangles are not joined at the end but are of 'open type' to facilitate increase or reduction in their diameter according to the requirement. In the megalith from where bangles and rings have been recovered, normally, iron objects of defence/attack have not been found. Such objects were probably confined to female burials only.

Gold

Two gold rings were found. One is of single coil, 'closed type' while the other is of 'open end' wire type spiral ear ring. They are in very pure form. They were found from the Megalith F. 2 from different levels.

Silver

One small ear ring of silver was also recovered form Megalith A. 2.

Bead

One broken barrel shaped stone bead (limestone) was recovered from Megalith B. 2.

Karkabhat, the nucleus

Location of hundreds of menhirs, cap-stones, cairn circles in the region of Karkabhat-Dhanora, spread over an area of nearly 5 sq. km. and complete absence of any other such concentration west of Mahanadi, in an area of at least 50 sq. km. shows that Karkabhat-Dhanora, due to its ideal location, easy accessibility, plenty of water and raw material for shaping and erecting megaliths, served as a nucleus point for performing the last rites of the departed whose mortal remains were disposed of either by cremation or by some other means. In the absence of any skeletal remains and burials in the area for which Karkabhat served as a nucleus point, cremation seems to be the most probable way. It was not necessary to erect these memorials immediately after the death of the person, these could be erected even later, when there used to be collective gathering at Karkabhat, depending on various religious, social and economic factors. There must have been a central religious authority to decide and declare the dates and control the whole affair. A similar parallel is found amongst one of the tribes in Bastar today who erect memorial stones at one particular spot. This function was organised in May-June 1991 after a gap of nearly twenty five years, when people even from Maharashtra also participated and after elaborate religious rites, erected memorial stones in honour of the departed ones, who left this world even twenty five years back.

Another Nucleus area

During the course of exploration when excavations at Karkabhat was in progress another Megalithic nucleus area of Karkabhat dimension was located east of Mahanadi on its right bank at Aroud-Lilar-Bhwanmara area. Here also, like Karkabhat area, hundreds of megaliths and cairn circles of all varieties are available. A survey of nearly 50 sq. km. of area east of Mahanadi in this region did not reveal any other megalithic remains. It appears that Arond-Lilar-Bhawanmara area served as a nucleus area for megalithic people, east of Mahanadi.

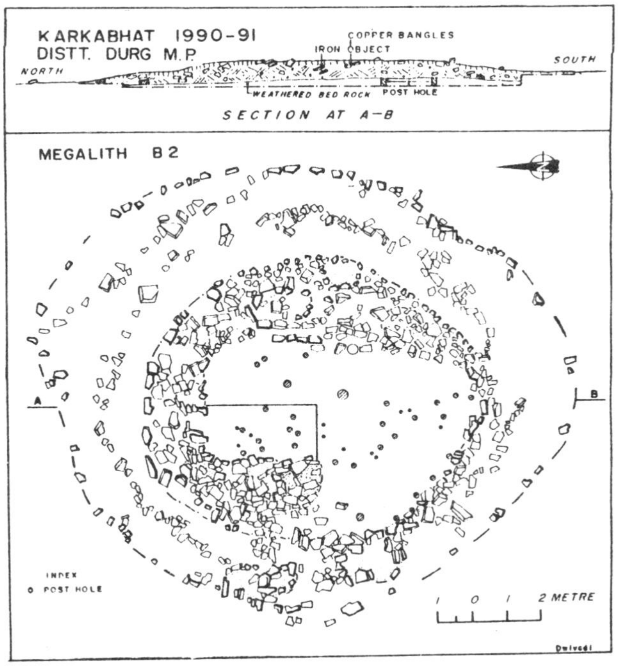

Dating

So far no dates are available for megalithic period in Chattisgarh region. On the basis of complete iron tool typology, megalithic remains at Karkabhat could be dated to around 1st half of first millennium B.C.

The Sculptured Menhir

The most startling and important find was the sculptured menhir*. The sculpted menhir has been put in the centre of cairn heap (pl. XII). Above the cairn heap the available height of the menhir is 2.57 m. and width is 1.91 m. It has been erected in perfect north-south position, i.e. widthwise east-west with the finished surface looking to the north and sculpted edge towards east. The masterly stroke of the sculptor has brought out a magnificent facial view of a man having receding broad forehead, with prominent glabella point, sharp long nose, broad and prominent ridge in the upper lip below nasal spine, pronounced lower lip and protruded chin. On the northern face eye has also been carved out. In the absence of chisel marks it is at the moment difficult to find out the type of tool or tools used by the master sculptor to prepare the grand profile.

REFERENCES

Gururaja Rao, B.K. 1972. *Megalithic Culture in South India.* Mysore University of Mysore.

Indian Archaeology 1956-57 *A Review.* 1956-57. New Delhi. Archaeological Survey of India: 35.

Rizvi, S.A. (Ed.) 1981. *Uttar Pradesh District Gazetteers.* Lucknow. Govt of Uttar Pradesh.

Sundara, A. 1979. Typology of Megaliths in South India. In *Essays in Indian Protohistory.* D.P. Agrawal & D.K. Chakrabarti (Ed.). Delhi.

* This is the opinion of the author - Editor

Inscribed Copper Tablets from Mohenjo-daro: Some Observations

B.M. PANDE*

In a paper (Pande 1973) published some years ago, we had attempted an analysis of the inscribed copper tablets from Mohenjo-daro bringing out certain facts peculiar to them. For instance, it was seen that in most if not all cases, certain inscriptions in the copper tablets generally have particular reverse device.[1] This however cannot be said to be the rule since there are also two different inscriptions (Nos. 10, 11, 89; and Nos. 70, 71, 72, 73)[2] with the same animal figure on the reverse or few examples of inscription on the obverse having different device on the reverse (Nos. 8, 9; 29, 30, 31, 32, 33, 34; 16, 79, 80; and 64, 65, 66, 67). Notwithstanding these shall we say, aberrations - it was obvious that there is some correspondence between the inscription on the obverse of the copper tablets and the device on the reverse. This was in contra-distinction to the inscriptions in other media, particularly the seals and sealings, where there does not seem to exist such a correspondence or connection between the inscription and the figure, symbol or device occurring alongwith it. Another distinct feature of the copper tablets is that the inscription engraved on each tablet is single-lined and in the few examples where there is a second line (Nos. 6, 7, 61, 73) it seems to have been added subsequently. Examples of inscription occurring alongwith the figure on the reverse side are only two (Nos. 14, 112). Of the two inscriptions, the inscription on the reverse of No. 14 comprising three signs is found in No. 3, where it occurs alongwith two more signs: it is thus obvious that the inscription on the obverse of No. 3 comprises of two blocks. In one case only there seems to be engraved in a corner above the animal figure on the reverse what appears to be a doubtful Harappan sign and is rather to be ignored (No. 114).

Equally important is the fact that these copper tablets are found only at Mohenjo-daro and this is quite significant. In fact, these copper tablets present a few other singular features which are absent in the other inscribed material from other Harappan sites. These features peculiar to the copper tablets comprise certain figures or symbols which occur on one face and which are not seen in the other inscribed material either from Mohenjo-daro or other Harappan sites. The figures which are engraved on the reverse of the copper tablets and are exclusive to them are: animal with two heads, one at either end of the body[3] (Nos. 10, 11, 70, 71, 72, 73, 89); hare[4] (Nos.

* Archaeological Survey of India, Janpath, New Delhi.

Paper read at the seminar organized by the Bihar Puravid Parishad, Patna, 18-19 October, 1986.

50, 51, 52, 53, 54, 55, 92, 111 and 119); horned archer[5] (Nos. 31, 32, 33); endless knot motif[6] (Nos. 61, 62, 63 and 91); and double axe.[7] The inscription on the obverse of the copper tablets which goes with the two-headed animal figure on the reverse is not common in all cases as already pointed out above. Out of the seven specimens, three (Nos. 10, 11, 89) contain the inscription 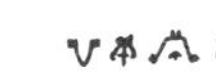 while the inscription on the other four (Nos. 70, 71, 72, 73) is 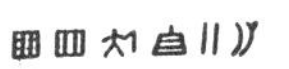 One of these (No. 73) has an additional line which is clearly a later addition; the inscription comprising the additional line is, 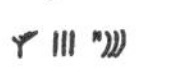 .[8] We can thus say that the inscriptions 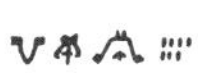 and 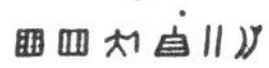 are connected with this figure. These inscriptions, including the additional line in Sl. No. 73 are not repeated in any other media nor is the animal, as already stated, found in the seals or sealings.

The inscription 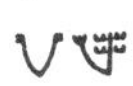 in No. 1 is, again, a lone specimen.[10] These two signs on the obverse of this copper tablet however recur in combination with two signs in No. 2 which has on its reverse chimeric figure of an elephant with horns.[11]

The combination of signs in No. 3 forming the inscription 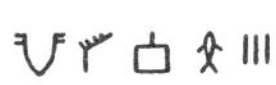 on the reverse is again unique to it even though the block 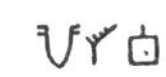 occurs as an inscription on the obverse of the copper tablet, No. 14 where it occurs alongwith the figure of goat-antelope.[12]

In all the copper tablets containing the figure of the hare on one face has the same inscription 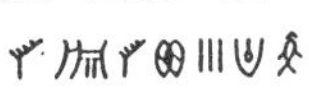 thereby indicating that the inscription is connected with this figure. This is further attested to by the fact that this inscription is also not repeated in the inscriptions in other media.[13] Incidentally, of the eleven occurrences of the sign 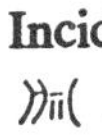 , which is juxtaposed with the sign 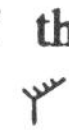 on its either side in the copper tablets, ten are on copper tablets.[14]

It was also seen that certain Harappan signs which occur on one face of some of the copper tablets as solus signs are not found in the other inscribed media. These signs are  ,  , 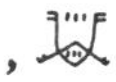 , 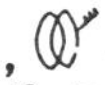 , having respectively 2, 3, 2 and 1 occurrences.[15] In both the copper tablets which have the sign  on oneface, the inscription is 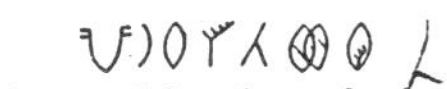 It is interesting to note that this inscription also occurs in copper tablets having the horned archer on one face. Could we, then, seek some connection between the sign and the horned archer? Copper tablets containing the sign 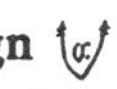 on one face have two types of inscriptions on the other face which is 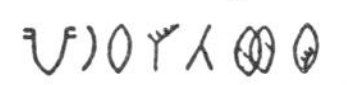 and 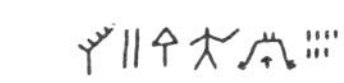 While the former inscription also occurs, as already pointed out above, with the sign  and horned archer, the latter is found in copper tablets having the goat antelope on the other face. The inscription on the obverse of the copper tablets containing the sign 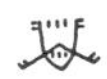 is 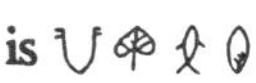 which is also found on copper tablets having the figure of an animal looking backwards.[16] Finally, the inscription on the copper tablet containing the sign  is also peculiar to it.

In sum, it is evident that there is some correspondence between the inscription on the copper tablets with either the symbol, sign or the animal or human figure on the other face. Likewise, it is also seen that the inscriptions occurring on the copper tablets are peculiar to them and are not found in the inscriptions in other media.

As already pointed out in our earlier paper, the inscriptions on copper tablets were not used as seals for stamping purposes and are therefore to be read as engraved (the only exceptions being Sl. Nos. 9, 67, 75 where the inscriptions have been reversed perhaps due to scribe's error).[17]

What then could have been the purpose and use of the copper tablets? The fact that these are confined only to Mohenjo-daro is indicative of their restricted use. So also is the singularity in terms of obvious relationship and connection between the inscription and the figure, symbol or sign, most of which, again, are found only in copper tablets. The use of metal for this class of objects in contrast to the other inscribed material also bespeaks of their importance.

Is it that these copper tablets were prized possessions of the important or dominant group of families of Mohenjo-daro and the figure or symbol on one face represents the totemic symbol or insignia[18] of each of these and were passed from generation to generation in the same family? Those of the copper tablets which contain an additional line which, as already stated above, was not originally meant, had perhaps changed hands from one family to another which added its inscription to make this change.

The copper tablets being restricted to Mohenjo-daro alone, the exclusivity of the field symbols and their limited number could perhaps be due to the fact that these belonged to and were the family or guild tokens[19] of the dominant group of families of Mohenjo-daro who - if we may hypothesize — were controlling the vast area covered by the Harappans.

NOTES

[1] As in our earlier paper (Pande 1973), the face of the copper tablet containing the inscription was called by us as obverse while the reverse has an animal or human figure or a symbol. The numbers referred to are the same as given in our earlier paper where we had included 123 copper tablets. However, Iravatham Mahadevan (1977) has included 135 copper tablets.

[2] These numbers refer to the serial number of copper tablets given in our earlier paper (Pande 1973). Unless otherwise stated, the numbers referred to are the ones given in our earlier paper.

[3] This corresponds to Field Symbol No. 29 of Mahadevan (1977, p. 794, pl. III, fig. No. 56). He describes it as a 'Fabulous animal of uncertain description with two heads, one at either end of the body'. Mahadevan has listed nine occurrences of this animal, all on copper tablets from Mohenjo-daro; cf. Tables VIII and IX.

[4] Mahadevan (1977, p. 793, pl. III, fig. No. 42), Field Symbol No. 16: 'hare facing a bush'. Mahadevan has listed eleven examples all of which occur on the copper tablets.

[5] Mahadevan (1977, p. 795, pl. V, fig. No. 89). Field Symbol No. 52: 'Standing personage with horns and bovine features, holding a bow in one hand and an arrow or an uncertain object in the other'. Mahadevan has listed six occurrences of this figure, all from Mohenjo-daro and occurring only on copper tablets, *vide* his Tables VIII and IX.

[6] Mahadevan (1977, p. 796, pl. VI, fig. No. 124), Field Symbol No. 86.

[7] Mahadevan (1977, p. 797, pl. VII, fig. No. 133), Field Symbol No. 95. 'Double-axe (?) without shaft'. According to Mahadevan, there is only one example of this field symbol which is on a copper tablet from Mohenjo-daro. The copper tablet containing this motif or symbol is in the collection of the Archaeological Survey of India bearing No. 63.10.419 and is not included in our earlier paper.

[8] In our earlier paper (Pande, 1973) the inscription is not clear and we have copied it from Mahadevan (1973: 94. Texts. No. 3347).

[9] M ahadevan 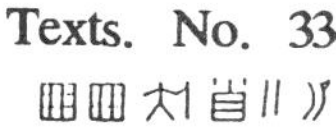

[10] In Mahadevan (1977, No. 2921), the inscription is given as 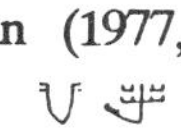 and the obverse sign as ||||| in the original, the lines are obliquely engraved and are not vertical.

[11] Mahadevan (1977, p. 794), Field Symbol No. 25. 'Fabulous animal with the body of a ram, horns of a bull, trunk of an elephant, hindlegs of a tiger and an upraised serpent-like tail'. Out of the twenty examples listed by Mahadevan, 18 are from Mohenjo-daro and 1 each from Harappa and Lothal. This figure on the copper tablet is a lone example.

[12] Mahadevan (1977, p. 793), Field Symbol No. 13.

[13] Mahadevan (1977, p. 710). In our earlier paper we had published 9 examples while Mahadevan has included 11 examples, all of which carry the same inscription and figure respectively on the obverse and the reverse.

[14] Mahadevan, 1977, Table IV.

[15] Mahadevan, 1977, Table IV.

[16] Mahadevan has called this figure also as goat-antelope (Field Symbol No. 13).

[17] Pande, 1973, p. 306.

[18] Ratnagar (1981: 246-249) has also suggested that the field symbols represent the totemic symbols or insignia or lineage emblems of the owners. Her hypothesis is amply attested to by the evidence of copper tablets where there is a clear connection between the inscription and the field symbol.

[19] The use of the copper tablets 'as authentic tokens in commercial transactions' suggested by us (Sarkar and Pande, 1969-70, p. 47) elsewhere may perhaps not be correct. In this paper we had also suggested 'their use as family or guild tokens.'

REFERENCES

Mahadevan, Iravatham. 1977. *The Indus Script: Texts, Concordance and Tables,* Memoirs of the Archaeological Survey of India. 77. New Delhi.

Pande, B.M. 1973. Inscribed copper tablets from Mohenjo-daro: a preliminary analysis. *Radiocarbon and Indian Archaeology.* Bombay: 305-322. Also reprinted in Gregory L. POSSEHL, *Ancient Cities of the Indus.* New Delhi. Vikas Publishing House Ltd. 1979: 268-283.

Ratnagar, Shereen. 1981. *Encounters: The Westerly Trade of the Harappa Civilization.* Delhi. Oxford University Press.

Sarkar, H. and B.M. Pande. 1969-70. A note on a knot design from Mohenjo-daro and its occurrence in later times. *Puratattva.* 3.

LIST OF HARAPPAN INSCRIPTIONS/SIGNS OCCURRING IN THE PAPER

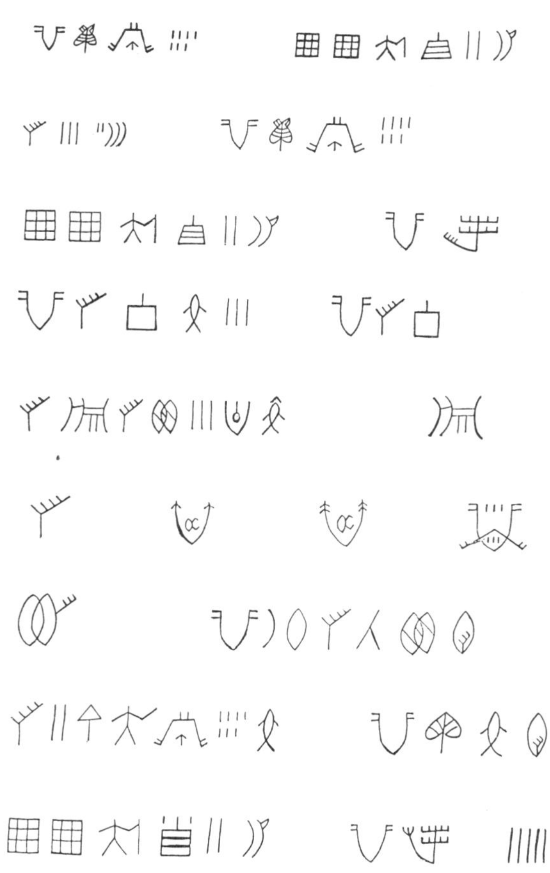

Beginning of Iron Age in Garhwal, Mid-Central Himalaya: An Ecological Overview

VINOD NAUTIYAL, K.P. NAUTIYAL, B.M. KHANDURI, D.L. RAJPUT*

INTRODUCTION

The studies on Iron Age and its beginning in the Indian sub-continent have been a widely discussed subject. Investigations of the last few decades have yielded valuable data on its various facets (Agrawal 1982; Allchin and Allchin 1982; Banerjee 1965; Bharadwaj 1976; Chakrabarti 1973a, 1973b, 1976, 1983, 1984-85; Ghosh 1973, 2976, Hegde 1976; Kosambi 1963; Lal 1954-55; Lal, M. 1984, 1986; Sahi 1982, 1987, 1989; Tripathi 1973, 1976). On the basis of its distribution pattern in India and adjoining areas Chakrabarti (1976, 1983) identified six iron-bearing foci with different cultural sub-stratum spread widely over from Baluchistan in the North-West to the Indo-Gangetic divide and the Ganga-Yamuna Doab in the north extending eastward and further South.

There is a general consensus that the introduction of iron did play a crucial role in changing the economic base of the settlers in the Ganga-Yamuna Doab, which formed the northern-most extension of the Iron Age culture in the Indian sub-continent (Banerjee, 1965; Chakrabarti 1973a, 1976; Tripathi, 1976). Obviously such assumption is significant and further extends the limit of the Iron Age culture to extreme north reaching right into the mid-Central Himalayan region of Garhwal and Kumaun. This region in its own way claims to be an important area of this culture, though so far placed in a complete cultural vacuum from the protohistoric time to the early historical period. With such meagre evidence attempts were scarcely made to study the Iron Age culture in the mid-Central Himalaya comprising Garhwal and Kumaun. In this connection a few passing references to the region are notable, particularly regarding the age-old existing Copper and Iron mines. They were supposed to have been exploited by an indigenous technology, first during the Copper Hoard Culture and later at the advent of the Iron Age in the Ganga-Yamuna Doab (Banerjee, 1965; Agrawal, 1982; Lal, 1984). Nevertheless, on the basis of archaeological investigations in recent years an altogether different picture has emerged for this area. Consequently, this has disproved an earlier belief of its being a cultural non-entity. In the light of new results it is now possible to say that the mid-Central Himalaya like the rest of the Indian sub-continent had also witnessed an emergence and expansion of early human societies around the beginning and later half of the first millennium B.C. practicing iron metallurgy (Nautiyal and Khanduri, 1977; Nautiyal 1982; Nautiyal and Khanduri 1986). These findings from this part have enlarged our scope for studying the Iron Age culture in a broader perspective adding new data in an Indian contextual framework. Consequently in view of the above, we observe that the so called scheme of grouping of six or four early Iron using centres in India needs to be revised along with the mid-Central Himalayan region exclusive of the parameter of the Ganga-Yamuna Doab.

* Department of Ancient Indian History, Culture And Archaeology, H.N.B. Garhwal University, Srinagar, Garhwal, U.P. 246 174.

In understanding the beginning of iron technology followed by its dispersal and subsequent impact on the process of urbanization in mountainous landscape, we are bound to take into consideration the various parameters, such as the distribution and history of mining and development of iron technology in their different ecological zones and impact on local landscape.

Ecological and Cultural Context of Iron Technology: An Altitudinal Profile

The landscape of mid-Central (Garhwal) Himalaya (Long 77° 49,′ 80° 6′ - Lat 29° 28′ - 39° 28′ N) due to altitudinal variation provides a series of geologic, geomorphic vegetative traits and therefore, a corresponding climatic zonation. Ranging from the sub-montane in the foothills of lesser Himalayas to montane in the middle river valleys and a sub-alpine and alpine in the high altitude regions. It is in these diverse ecological zones that the following three different cultures developed, from the beginning of the first millennium B.C. till the beginning of the Christian era, evolving their own smelting technologies.

(i) Megalithic cave burial culture datable to c. 1000 B.C. in the high altitude alpine zone.
(ii) Protohistoric to early and late historical cultures datable between c. 1000 B.C. to c. A.D. 1100. in the lower altitude in the river valleys
(iii) Early and a late historical settlement in the foothills of the mid-Central Himalaya (The Tarai and Bhabar belt) datable between c. 500 B.C. to 2nd century A.D.
(iv) Iron tools in an ethnoarchaeological framework found in a very unconventional context embedded in the trunk of a modern oak *(Quercus semicarphifolia)* tree in the sub-alpine zone at Bhekal Tal in district Chamoli.

HIGH ALTITUDE ZONE (ALPINE AND SUB-ALPINE)

The alpine zone is characterised by a dominant and widespread grassland, birch forest, silver fir and junipers reflecting a xerophytic type of vegetation. The xerophytic character which developed in plants at high altitude is due to certain climatic factors like scarcity of soil moisture, high wind velocity high aridity and thin soil cover (Purohit 1977). It is because of these climatic factors in the high altitude alpine zone that the cultivation of traditional crops like wheat, barley and rice is not prevalent on a large scale as a regular crop. Consequently, the present day inhabitants cultivate a few crops like potato, phapar *(Fagopyrum lataricum) Ogal, (Fagopyrum esculantum), Mandua (Elucine coracana),* etc. (Gaur 1982).

Before discussing the emergence of iron technology in high altitude, it is essential to understand the cultural background of the Iron Age settlers in that particular region. The archaeology of high altitude in the mid-Central Himalaya, if compared to the Trans-Himalaya, is not well documented because of the paucity of archaeological data from the inhospitable geographical zone. However, in the high altitude region of mid-Central Himalaya and nearer the western border of Tibet a few earlier workers had reported a few megalithic burials (Henwood 1858; Wheeler 1959) recalling a similar burial tradition in the whole of Himalayan range consisting of the region of Kashmir, Ladakh (Francke 1914) Lahul and Chamba in district Kangra (Sankrityayan 1953) including a major part of north western India (Dani 1967) and Swat in Pakistan (Silvi Antonini and Stacul, 1972). This area bearing cultural remnants of the first millennium B.C. was anciently designated as the Gandhara region. Recently the problem has received a fresh assessment particularly in relation to the genesis of the burial culture in the Garhwal-Kumaon region (Bhatt and Nautiyal 1988; Nautiyal 1989). On the basis of literary and archaeological findings, they have also associated the graves of mid-Central Himalayan region of Garhwal to a homogeneous group of tribes of the Khasas, Dards, Abhisaras, Tanganas, Kiratas who had settled widely in the mid-Central Himalaya after traversing a long migration route from their original home in Central Asia (Nautiyal and Khanduri 1986). It is now by our latest investigations that the evidence of ancient human settlement in the alpine zone has been recorded in a definite manner. Primarily, we have at present an evidence of horse burial complex at Malari (IAR 1984-85).

The site of Malari (Lat. 70° 50′ N, Long. 79° 55′ 50") is situated at an altitude of 3500 m. in district Chamoli, about 63 km. north-east of Josimath on way to Niti Pass. Here a series of burials have been reported earlier. In our earlier communication we have preferred to designate these caves with skeletal remains as a burial complex (IAR 1984-85), but on our later investigation of a self-exposed cave at Malari with inter-connected chambers, we are inclined to amend and say that besides disposing of the dead, the mountain dwellers simultaneously utilized such chambers for their purpose. While excavating one of such cave burials, we found skeletal remains of a horse along with large-sized black and red slipped jars placed all around the animal skeleton. They are painted in white pigment with horizontal and vertical lines. At times there are grooved lines subsequently filled up with red and white colour (Fig. 2). A few of the spouted vessels are showing a clear-cut Central Asiatic affiliation (Grishman 1952).

In addition to these the discovery of a variety of large number of highly fragile iron implements is significant. Most of the implements, though weather-worn, include such shapes as the arrowhead, chisel, barbed arrowhead, rings and rectangular chunks of iron with some impressions. Out of them, a few iron nails measuring approximately 5-7 cm. in length deserve special mention (Fig. 3). A careful examination of these implements indicates that the thin hard twigs of oak were pierced with drill from one end to the other so as to easily insert the thin iron nails in them. This seems to have been achieved after heating up the iron nails to a maximum degree and driving them easily into these wooden twigs. The frontal end of the nail was sharpened and pointed. This proves that the inhabitants at this altitude had evolved a kind of specialized technique to manufacture these iron implements particularly for hunting purpose.

Though precise function of these interesting implements of Malari is simply a matter of speculation at present, yet it is quite logical to assume that the wooden shielding was intentionally done to manipulate the dynamics of these tiny nails or arrowheads for hunting small preys, like birds or other small animals.

Thus the indications are not wanting to assume that the Malari inhabitants were extensively using iron implements for hunting. The smelting of iron, however, was not practised by them as no iron slags and evidence of hearth remains have been found inside the dwelling chambers. The observation that smelting was done probably elsewhere but nearer the area finds support from the fact that the old working mine at Siyasain which is less than 20 km. NW of Malari, was a rich iron-ore site, as mentioned before.

On account of the absence of any plant or seed remains from the burial complex, it is difficult to reconstruct the subsistence pattern of these settlers. Keeping in view the climatic stresses of the high altitude region the iron implements may not have been sufficiently useful for any kind of agricultural practice. This is more or less clear that the beginning of agriculture in the Himalayas was restricted only to north western valleys, as reported from early Neolithic levels of Burzahom and in the aceramic Neolithic level at Gofkral in Kashmir (Mittre 1977; Sharma 1982). However, it was comparatively a late phenomenon in such a high altitude terrain, where it would have been more difficult to cut the mountain slopes for making narrow terraces. On such indications we may assume that hunting and pastoral activity have been the main source of livelihood at Malari. It may also be added that since iron implements along with pottery became an important mainstay they assumed special significance (pls. XIII-XIV).

The chronology of this settle-cum burial complex cannot be finally established. But on the basis of pottery along with iron, it has been tentatively placed in c. 1000 B.C.

TEMPERATE ZONE

In contrast to the xerophytic vegetation of the Alpine zone, the vegetation of the temperate zone is characterised by a mixed deciduous type of flora dominated by Kharsu Oak *(Querus semicarpifolia)*, Burans *(Rhododendron arboreum)*, Bhojpatra *(Betula utilis)*, Maple *(Acer caesium)* and Fir *(Abis pindro)*. The climate of this zone is humid with high rainfall and due to this a good soil cover has developed here. Kharakwal (1977) ascribes this soil type as a brown deciduous and grey forest soil which is good for cultivation.

It is in this ecological zone that several high altitude glacial lakes are situated in Garhwal Himalaya (Prasad and Sundriyal 1986). Bhaikal Tal (Long. 29° 35′ E, Lat. 30° 8′ N) which was taken up for an archaeological investigation, is one of such perennial lakes situated at an altitude of 3000 m. and located amidst a thick forest of Oak *(Quercus semicarpifolia)* about 40 km west of Gwaldam in district Chamoli. Due to rich meadows and grassland environs the area is favourable for transhumance, but agricultural activities are only confined to the lower altitude of this zone. It was also revealed that agricultural practices mainly rested on potato cultivation and a few other cereals, which make a staple diet even for the present day populace.

Since Bhaikal Tal is located in the midst of a thick forest, it has been ideally suited for temporary settlement during the months of summer when the Himalayan meadows attract herdsmen from the foothills and also from the middle region of the Himalaya. Therefore, with a view to find out the earlier evidence of such a transhumance settlement, investigation was conducted in the area around the lake in 1986. Although exploration and a trial excavation subsequent upon it at various spots did not yield fruitful results, yet an interesting aspect, the dried-up lake where a large number of arrowheads were found embedded on the truck of the two oak

(Quercus semicarpifolia) trees, was recorded here.

The following four different categories of iron implements with minor variations were recorded (Fig. 4).

(A) Arrowhead showing an equal length of body and working edge

(a) with a square cut top;
  (i) With thick upper portion of the body, thick tail with broken end;
  (ii) with sharply cut profile equal on all the sides;

(b) With rounded top;
  (i) small in size, tail merging with the body but almost similar to the above.

(B) Arrowhead with an elongated body and a small tail

(a) Elongated body with a sharply cut top portion appearing as a small tail (damaged);
(b) medium-sized, elongated body with tail ranging from 1 cm. to 3 cm.;
(c) small-sized arrowhead with smaller body and tail;
  (i) with an elongated tail;
  (ii) with a smaller tail.

(C) Elongated body and sharply pointed tail

(a) less flat with prominent mid-rib;
(b) less flat with tail merging with the body of the spearhead, mid-rib slightly prominent;
(c) same as above, but with elongated body, mid-rib unmodified;
(d) less flat than (i) and the tail merging with the body.

Taking into consideration the morphological and topological features of these implements, particularly the arrowheads, it can be admitted that these are comparable with the iron arrowheads of Ranihat datable to c. 5th cent. B.C. Though there is a very large time gap between the two groups of iron implements, yet the Bhaikal Tal collection belonging roughtly to c. 17th-18th cent. A.D. shows a continuity of the older tradition of Ranihat, particularly in shape and size.

A close observation of the context of the implements at Bhaikal Tal indicates that these were probably deliberately nailed into the tree trunks by some human agency in respect of a kind of religious totem or as part of some village ritual, which no longer exists in the area.

Based on an ethnoarchaeological evidence from Bhaikal Tal, it can be presumably be said that the tradition of fabricating iron implements has continued in mid-Central Himalaya till the present times. This is more so for the inhabitants of this region might have exploited the local ores of Mok and Charbanga mines for smelting iron ore and manufacturing implements indigenously till a very recent time. Morphologically, such implements were basically required for smaller games and not for agriculture or any other purpose. Since the implements were basically life sustaining device for the people of high altitude zone, they were invariably worshipped in the temples and gained ritualistic significance.

River Valleys

The vegetation in the river valleys indicates a gradual variation in accordance with the elevation and topography. The vegetation comprises mixed temperate to tropical component reflecting varied climatic pattern, but the predominant feature of this zone is a moist tropical climate with low light intensity, higher temperature, low rainfall and low humidity. Therefore, owing to these ecological factors the soil cover is well developed for cultivating various crops.

During the remote past these factors might have facilitated the growth and expansion of ancient settlements in the river valleys. Lately, our preliminary investigations in the Bhagirathi and the Bhilangana river valleys have shown that the frequency of the early and late historical settlements is higher in this zone as compared to the alpine and temperate zone. The excavation at Thapli (Nautiyal et al. 1981), Ranihat (Nautiyal and Khanduri 1977) and Purola (Nautiyal and Khanduri 1988-89) in the Alaknanada and the Kamal valleys have confirmed our hypothesis that this zone was prone to cross cultural influences and was continuously inhabited by ancient settlers right from protohistoric period onwards.

But so far as the beginning of iron technology is concerned, it may be pointed out that unlike the Ganga-Yamuna Doab, where the iron technology started around the first millennium B.C. we do not have any definite indicator to say when the local mines were first exploited and tools were made thereof. This is not known even during the arrival of the PGW users in the river valleys of mid-Central Himalaya. The Thapli and Purola results are silent about the same. Assuming, therefore a late beginning we can say that the iron technology here was a phenomenon of c. 5th cent. B.C., when there was an advent of the early historical settlers at Ranihat (Nautiyal and Khanduri 1977). The causes of this belated arrival of iron in the Himalayan river valleys cannot be explained in the light of the present available archaeological data. However, we can deduce two plausible explanations.

(a) That the PGW culture at Thapli and Purola belongs to the formative stages of the expansion of one group of Aryans in the Drishdavati valley (Gaur 1984) and at the same time to the Yamuna and the Ganga valleys. This period coincides with the pre-iron phase of the PGW culture similar to that of the early PGW phase identified at Bhagwanpura (Joshi 1978).

(b) The second possible centre may have been located in the Ganga Yamuna Doab and the Tarai belt of the foothills of lesser Himalaya. But interestingly, the archaeological evidence from the two excavated sites at Bharat Mandir in district Dehradun and Moradhwaj in district Bijnor clearly indicates that though the early settlement with mud-brick structure commenced around c. 5th cent B.C., yet iron was introduced here even later in the beginning of c. 2nd century B.C. (Nautiyal, et al. 1979) (Table 1).

In light of these evidences, it is possible to say that iron technology may not have arrived in the river valleys of mid-Central Himalaya from the foothll region, but rather from the high altitude zones, where it had reached around c. 1000 B.C. as indicated by the evidence at Malari.

Ranihat Evidence

It may also be pointed out that there is sufficient archaeological evidence to prove that around c 5th cent. B.C. the ancient settlers at Ranihat not only fabricated iron implements, but also carried out the technique of smelting iron ore within the habitational area (Nautiyal and Khanduri 1977, 1986). This is proved by the discovery of a round hearth along with iron slags at lowest level at Ranihat. In all probability the ancient settlers at Ranihat exploited the iron ore of Dhanpur and Pokhri. The iron tool repertoire includes several types of arrowheads, chisel, rings, knife, fishhooks, etc. (Fig. 5). The conspicuous absence of agricultural implements such as spade, sickle, hoe, axe and ploughshare from Ranihat makes it possible to 'infer the exact agricultural practices adopted by the permanent settlers at Ranihat, though it cannot be ruled out that the inhabitants did practice agriculture along with cultivation. It is obviously clear that due to a riverine habitat the inhabitants (c. 600 B.C. to c. A.D. 800 might considerably have depended on the available resources and carried fishing and hunting as a prominent source of their sustenance.

Sub-Tropical Zone (Bhabar and Tarai Belt)

The terms Tarai and Bhabar are applied to the broad belt of foothill country which separates the Siwalik and the Indo-Gangetic plain. This submontane zone thus consists of a characteristic post-tertiary depositional phenomenon.

The Bhabar, basically a belt of waterless forest is a zone of alluvial fan with porous sandy soil at the foot of the Siwalik range, extending from the Yamuna to the Sharda River covering an area of 8 to 20 sq. km in width. As no water rises from the gravel there is a thin covering of alluvial soil on its vast dry bed of boulders. The forest cover is extremely luxuriant here and derives moisture from the sub-soil. In sharp contrast to Bhabar, the Tarai zone lying south of Bhabar and north of the Ganga-Yamuna Doab and characterized by the presence of reed and grass indicated a marshy and swampy landform. On account of this feature Kalapesi (1980) has designated this zone as a "Humid Island" or "watr soaked land".

It is under this ecological background that the Bhabar-Tarai belt had witnessed an emergence of ancient settlements. There are several literary, historical and travelling accounts providing sufficient details on the cultural history of this region (Atkinson 1882, Watters 1973, Cunningham 1975). Hieun Tsang (c. A.D. 629) provides a brief account of the then prevailing prolific settlements in the foothills of lesser HImalaya, particularly at Kashipur and Moradhwaj (Watters 1973, Cunningham 1924). In recent years the archaeological excavations have not only substantiated the available literary data, but have added a new dimension for understanding the nature and development of early and late historical settlements in the Bhabar and Tarai belt (Nautiyal et al. 1979).

Before discussing the advent and impact of iron technology in this zone, we shall briefly discuss the cultural sequence of Moradhwaj and Bharat Mandir; for this has a direct bearing to the beginning of iron technology in this region. The excavation at Moradhwaj puts the beginning of the early settlement around c. 5th century B.C. coinciding with he arrival of the Northern Black Polished Ware Culture (NBP) group in this belt, who raised burnt brick structures with mud-rampart wall. The occupation at Moradhwaj continued till c. 3rd-4th century A.D. The most notable feature, apart from building activity and ceramic tradition, was the development and perfection of terracotta art, which flourished during the early

Kushana period (Nautiyal et al. 1979). Similarly, the earliest occupation at Bharat Mandir commenced around the second century B.C., with the same ceramic tradition of Moradhwaj. The structural activity in both sites continued unabated until the late Kushana period (c. 3rd-4th cent. A.D.) but at Bharat Mandir it was occupied once again after a gap of five centuries.

The excavations at both sites have also highlighted that the foothill of Garhwal Himalaya remained a thriving centre for a permanent occupation continuously for at least seven or eight hundred years. Since this region formed a peripheral zone of the Ganga-Yamuna Doab, the cultural milieu in the Bhabar-Tarai belt in all probability was strongly influenced by the NBP phase Iron-Age settlers of the Ganga-Yamuna Doab.

However, a complete absence of Iron implements from the earlier NBP and fine grey ware levels at these two sites is enigmatic in view of the fact that around c. 6th and 5th centuries B.C. iron technology had reached its zenith in the entire Indo-Gangetic plain, as revealed from the excavations of a few important sites like Hastinapur (Lal 1954, 55), Ahicchhatra, (Ghosh and Panigrahi 1946), Atranjikhera (Gaur 1984), Hulas, Dikshit, 1981) Allhapur (Dikshit, 1973), and Kaushambi (Sharma 1987). This development not only formed an important cultural segment of the society but also brought a stability in agricultural productions (Sahi 1982). In contrast to this the situation seems to be totally different in the Bhabar-Tarai zone where the iron metallurgy seems to have emerged only around c. 2nd cent. B.C and gradually proliferated in the beginning of Christian era. This is clear from the frequency table which shows a sharp increase in the total number of different implements in period II B at Moradhwaj and Period I B and II at BHarat Mandir, corresponding to the late phase of occupation at both the site (Table 1).

Taking into consideration the ecological constraints of the Tarai-Bhabar zone, we can only make some broad generalizations. In this regard we may hypothesize that the ecology of this zone during the second half of the first millennium B.C. may not have been favourable for agricultural practice due to its marshy and swampy conditions. On account of these conditions, it is quite likely that the inhabitants during the early phase of occupation had remained grossly dependent for cereals and other food resources upon their neighbouring population of the Ganga-Yamuna Doab where early urban centers had emerged and the advent of the two-wheeled-chariot had facilitated the movement of people and goods (Sahi 1987). This practice of procuring cereals may have persisted even during the late phase of the settlemnt. But due to the gradual population pressure on the Tarai-Bhabar belt it might have become difficult to sustain on the import of cereals from the main centers of the Ganga-Yamuna Doab. Besides, the quantum of cereals and other eatables might not have been sufficient to support the large population of foothills. This pressure coupled with the scarcity must have compelled the inhabitants to start the practise of shifting cultivation along with hunting in the peripheral zone of Bhabar and Tarai. It is quite likely that due to this requirement agricultural iron implements like sickles and chisels had come into use here around the beginning of the Christian era (Fig. 6).

Conclusion

The foregoing discussion proves beyond doubt that in contrast to the earlier-held belief, the Iron Age culture did extend to the peripheral zone beyond the Ganga-Yamuna Doab, i.e. towards the mid-Central Himalaya. The present study conclusively indicates that the iron technology in the mid-Central Himalaya was not linked organically with the nuclear zone of the Ganga-Yamuna Doab, but had formed an individual independent cultural entity, which stretched from the high altitude to the foothills of the Tarai-Bhabar belt. The genesis of Iron Age in the mid-Central Himalaya would still remain problematic until a firm and datable cultural horizon is excavated in the region. However, as the present evidence stands, it may be said that the iron technology in the high altitude developed independently not absolutely because of any external stimulus, but also due to availability of local rich iron ore, which facilitated the activity.

REFERENCES

Agrawal, D.P. 1982. The Archaeology of India. Scandinavian institute of Asian Studies Monograph series. 46.

Agrawal D.P. and A. Ghosh (Ed.) *Radio-carbon and Indian archaeology*. Tata Institute of Fundamental Research Bombay: 391-400.

Bhatt and Nautiyal. 1987-88. Trans Himalayan Burials, Vis-a-Vis Malari : An Assessment. JOHSARD. 11 & 12: 95-101.

Chakrabarti, Dilip, K. 1973a. Beginning of iron in India : Problems Reconstructed in A.K. Ghosh (Ed.) Perspective in palaeo-anthropology. Calcutta: 345-356.

Chakrabarti Dilip K., 1973b Beginning of iron and Social change in India. Indian Studies Past and Present. XIV: 329-38.

Chakrabarti, Dilip K. 1976. The beginning of iron in India. Antiquity. L: 114-124.

Chakrabarti, Dilip K. 1983. The issue of the Indian Iron Age (cyclostyled). Key paper in the Seminar on Recent advances in Indian Archaeology. Deccan College. Pune.

Chakrabarti, Dilip K. 1984-85. Iron and urbanization: An Examination of the Indian context. *Puratattva.* 15: 68-74.

Cunninggham, A. 1975. *Ancient Geography of India.* Delhi (Reprint).

Dani, A.H. 1967. Timargarh and Gandhara grave culture. *Ancient Pakistan.* III.

Dikshit, K.N. 1973. The Allhapur evidence and the PGW chronology in D.P. Agrawal and A. Ghosh (Ed.) *Radio-carbon and Indian Archaeology.* TIFR, Bombay: 148-157.

Dikshit, K.N. 1981. Excavation at Hulas and further exploration of the Ganga-Yamuna Doab, *Man & Environment* 5. 70-76.

Francke, A.H. 1914. ASI, AR. (1910): 104-106.

Gaur, R.C. 1984. *Excavation at Atranjikhera.* Delhi.

Ghrishman, R. 1952. Iron. 30. Middlesex.

Ghosh, A. 1976. Foreword to *The Painted Grey Ware - An Iron Age Culture of Northern India* (Vibha Tripathi). Delhi.

Ghosh, A. and K.C. Panigarhi. 1946. The potteries of Ancient India, *Ancient India.* 1. Delhi: 37-55.

Ghosh, N.C. and R.P. Sharma, 1976. A Note on the Excavation at Virabhadra. *Puratattva.* 8: 180-81.

Hegde, K.T.M. 1976. Early stages of Metallurgy in India in D.P. Agrawal and A. Ghosh (Ed.) *Radio-carbon and Indian archaeology.* TIFR. Bombay: 401-05.

Henwood, W.J. 1958. Notice of the Rock-Bason at Deo (Devi) Dhoora near Almora in Upper India. ENPJ, N.S. IV.

Joshi, J.P. 1978. Interlocking of Late Harappan and Painted Gray Ware in the light of recent Excavation. *Man & Environment.* 2. Pune: 98-101

Kalapesi Dhun, M. 1980. Understanding Himalayan Ecology in *Studies in Himalayan Ecology and Development strategies* (Ed., T.V. Singh. New Delhi. 10-26.

Kharakwal, S.C. 1977. Geographic personality of Garhwal. The Himalaya. 1-1. Srinagar: 3-13.

Kosambi, D.D. 1963. The beginning of Iron Age in India, *Journal of Economic and Social history of Orient.* 6: 3099-318.

Lal, B.B. 1954-55. Excavation at Hastinapur and other exploration in the upper Ganga and Satluj basin, 1950-52. *Ancient India.* 10-11.

Lal, B.B. The painted Grey Ware culture. chapter XVIII. *History of the Civilization of Central Asia.* UNESCO.

Lal, Makkhan. 1984. Settlement History and Rise of Civilization in Ganga-Yamuna Doab from 500 B.C. 300 A.D. New Delhi.

Lal, Makkhan. 1986. Iron Tools, Forest clearance and urbanization in the Gangetic plain. *Man & Environment.* Pune: 83-90.

Nautiyal, K.P. 1989. Protohistoric India. New Delhi.

Nautiyal, K.P. and B.M. Khanduri, 1977. Ranihat and its Environs: Excavation of an early historical site in Garhwal. *The Himalaya* 1. Srinagar (Garhwal): 22-38

Nautiyal, K.P. 1980. Evidence of New Cultural element in the Lesser Himalayan region of Garhwal. An appraisal. *MADHU Recent researches in Indian archaeology and art history.* Delhi.

Nautiyal, K.P. and B.M. Khanduri. 1979. Cultural evolution in Himalayan Tarai of Garhwal : Assessment of an excavation at Moradhwaj. *Journal of Himalayan Studies and Regional Development.* 3. Srinagar: 23-38.

Nautiyal K.P., Khanduri, B.M., Nautiyal Vinod, And, D.L. 1981. Thapli. A PGW site in Garhwal. *Puratattva.* 10. New Delhi: 94.

Nautiyal, K.P. and B.M. Khanduri, 1986. New Cultural Dimension in the central Himalayan Region of Uttarakhand - An Archaeological Assessment ANNALI: 77-100.

Nautiyal, K.P. and B.M. Khanduri, 1988-89. Excavations of a Vedic Brick Altar at Purola, district Uttarkashi, Central Himalaya: *Puratattva* 19. New Delhi: 68-69.

Purohit, A.N. 1977. Exploratory Survey of florastic pattern in Garhwal Himalaya and a possible adaptibility mechanism. *The Himalaya.* Srinagar (Garhwal). 1: 14-21.

Roy, T.N. 1983. The Ganga Civilization. New Delhi.

Sahi, M.D.N. 1982. Origin and Direction of Dispersal of Painted Grey Ware. Hypothesis.

Sahi, M.D.N. 1987. Agricultural production during the early Iron Age, Essays in Ancient Indian Economic History. (Ed.) B. Chattopadhaya New Delhi.

Sahi, M.D.N. 1989. Role of Iron in Socio-Economic Change in Northern India-Jakhera a Case Study. *Studies in India Culture and Archarology.*

Sankrityayan, Rahul. 1953. *Himalay Parichay.* 1, Allahabad: 1, 49.

Silvi Antonini, C. and G. Stacul, 1972. The proto-Historic Grayeards of Swat (Pakistan) Part-I. Description of Graves and Finds. IsMEO. Reports and Memoirs. VII 1. Rome.

Sharma, A.K. 1981. Animal Bones From Gofkral-Evidence of Human and Non-human activity. *Puratattva* 12: 31-36.

Sharma, R.S. 1975-76. Archaeological tradition-The later Vedic phase of the Painted Grey Ware culture. *Puratattva.* 8. New Delhi: 63-67.

Sundriyal, R.R. 1983. Regional Geology of the area between Dhanpur Pokhari, Garhwal Himalaya with special reference to occurrence of ore deposits. unpublished thesis. Garhwal University.

Thapar, Romila. 1978. Puranic Lineage and archaeological data. *Puratattva* 8: 86-98.

Tripathi, Vibha, 1973. Introduction of iron in India in D.P. Agrawal and A. Ghosh (Ed.) *Radio-carbon and Indian archaeology.* Tata Institute of Fundamental research Bombay: 272-298.

Tripathi, Vibha. 1976. Painted Grey Ware: An Iron Age culture. Delhi.

Vishnu-Mittre. 1976. Changing Economy in Ancient India. *Origin of Agriculture.* Charles A. Reed (Ed.) Mouton Publishers. The Hague. Paris: 569-588.

Watters, Thomas. 1973. On Yuan Chwang's Travels in India. New Delhi (Reprint): 322-30.

Wheeler, R.E.M. 1959. Early India and Pakistan London.

Ceramics and Maritime Routes of India: New Evidence

I.K. SARMA*

In this paper** an attempt has been made to put forth the ceramic evidences documented from the archaeological contexts ranging in date from early Mauryan (3rd century B.C.) to late medieval periods (17th century A.D.) of Indian history with special emphasis on the maritime routes that linked the neighbouring countries of the East. Three major ceramic periods are suggested while classifying the available data which is vast and of varied nature.

I. *Pottery Associated With Early Buddhist Spread (Mauryan to the End of Ist Century B.C.):*

A diagnostic pottery called Northern Black Polished Ware (NBP) characterises the earliest phase of the Buddhist centres of North-East - Rājagṛha, Śrāvastī, Vaiśāli, Kauśāmbī, Ujjainī, Vidiśā (Sāñchī), Sarnath, Taxila, besides of course the Mauryan capital Pāṭaliputra. The rise of the *Mahājanapadas* (16-Repulican States), and new awakening after Buddha's preaching led to a total transformation in the cultural and religious set up of Ancient India. The NBP Ware is a deluxe ware used by the monks and royal houses alike for its excellence and endurance. It is of superfine Gangetic clay, well fired, thin sectioned, grey to reddish coloured with a mirror-like thin film-like polish.

The surface hues include the shades of golden, steel blue, black and silvery. The types are simple and mostly bowls, dishes sharply carinated handles, rarely cups and lids. The pottery was very precious and it appears, even if some parts had broken they were mended with copper pins or cross-dowels and reused (Figs: 1-2).

The profusion of this pottery with the early Buddhist centres of India is well known. The spread of Buddhist faith by monarchs like Aśoka led to its expanse to peninsular India. But the evidences from the most important Buddhist centres of coastal Āndhra, like Amarāvatī-Vaḍḍamānu (in Guntur District of A.P.) and Chebrolu have revealed that NBP reached these parts during the early Mauryan period (Sarma 1989) itself alongwith the Buddhist missionaries from the Magadha area. Aśoka Maurya in fact endowed the already existing *Mahāchaītya* at Amarāvatī, with a Pillar edict and railing of granite uprights and caused the first beautification to this *Mahāstūpa* which enshrined the *Śarīra dhātu:* of the Master. *Manjuśrīmūla Kalpa* clearly says: *Śrī Dhāñyakaṭaka chaītye Jinadhātu dharebhuvī"*

The prolific occurrence of NBP ware at the Amarāvatī Dharaṇikōta excavations (1974-75) in such early contexts has opened up fresh grounds for study. In recent years, apart from the above evidences from Dhānyakaṭaka *stūpa,* some sites along the coastal Tamilnadu have yielded precious evidences (Gurumurthy 1981). The NBP ware from *Korkai,* an ancient port town of the Pāṇḍyas, and more recently Alagankulam (1989) near Ramanathapuram yielded NBP bowls in association with Silver Punch-marked coins within early historical cultural assemblage of Mauryan date. It is of great significance to note that NBP ware and Punch-marked coins were reported from the earliest levels of some Buddhist sites where fortified

* Archaeological Survey of India, New Delhi.

** Paper read in the International Seminar held at Madras (20-21st De.c. 1990) sponsored by the ASI on the eve of the arrival of the ship Fulk-al-Salamah.

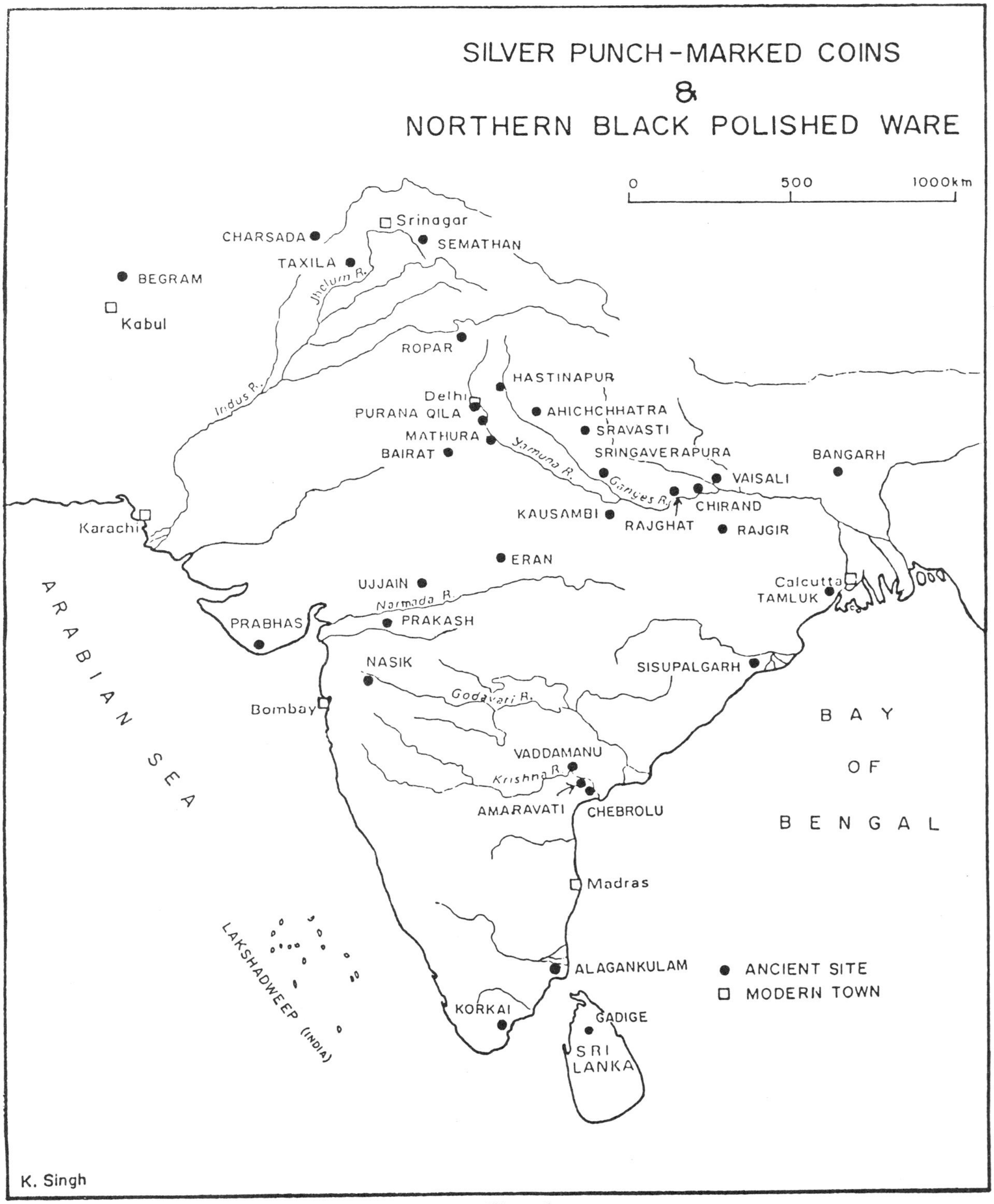
SILVER PUNCH-MARKED COINS
&
NORTHERN BLACK POLISHED WARE
0 500 1000km
Srinagar
CHARSADA
SEMATHAN
TAXILA
BEGRAM
Jhelum R.
Kabul
ROPAR
Indus R.
HASTINAPUR
Delhi
PURANA QILA
AHICHCHHATRA
SRAVASTI
MATHURA
BAIRAT
Yamuna R.
SRINGAVERAPURA
BANGARH
VAISALI
Ganges R.
CHIRAND
Karachi
KAUSAMBI
RAJGHAT
RAJGIR
ERAN
UJJAIN
Narmada R.
Calcutta
TAMLUK
ARABIAN SEA
PRABHAS
PRAKASH
NASIK
SISUPALGARH
Godavari R.
Bombay
BAY OF BENGAL
VADDAMANU
Krishna R.
AMARAVATI
CHEBROLU
Madras
LAKSHADWEEP (INDIA)
ALAGANKULAM
ANCIENT SITE
MODERN TOWN
KORKAI
GADIGE
SRI LANKA
K. Singh

Fig. 1

towns of Pre-Mauryan date (600-450 B.C.) were unearthed recently - specially Gedige and Anurādhapura citadel in Śrī Lanka (Deraniyagala 1986). In the light of these evidences, we may recall with profit the Buddhist legends enshrining certain important events. According to *Mahāvaṁśa* (XIV, 6 and XIX, 11-12) the Mauryan emperor Aśoka came to despatch the *Bodhivriksha* sapling to Siṁhala in a highly religious manner. He descended into water upto the neck and set the Bodhi tree on the ship (PL. 2) and stood with folded hands on the shore. Again *Mahāvaṁśa* narrates that King Dutthagamini of Śrī Lanka (101-77 B.C). celebrated with pomp the laying of great *stūpa* inviting many monks and kings from foreign lands (one *Mahādeva* from Pallava Bhogga and *Yona Mahādharmarakshita* from Alasandra (i.e. Alexandaria). The *Vinaya* texts and *Jātakas* inform us that merchants from Sahajati, Kauśāmbī, Vārāṇāsi, Pāṭalīputra and Gompa brought their goods to Tāmralipti (Tamluk, in Midnapore Dist. of West Bengal) for trade with South Asia. The sea port towns of great importance are Tāmralipti, (Gangae) and Kanthi on lower Bengal Coast, Kainapara (Konark), Dosarene (Dhauli, Orissa) Kalingae (Kalingapatnam) and Maisolia (Machilipatnam) in coastal Andhra. It is, therefore, becoming clear that the first ceramic viz. the N.B.P. ware with Punch-marked silver coins reached South-East Indian Port towns and farther beyond Śrī Lanka as well, by the end of 3rd Century B.C. along with the Buddhist monks and merchant guilds. *(Śreshṭhīs* and *Nigamas)* who were converts to this popular casteless religious faith.

The West Coast has a different story and till date no NBP/PMC or Buddhist monastic establishments of such magnitude and early date have been registered on the long Karnataka or Kerala coast line.

II. *Early Greek/Roman Impact : Pottery Wares and Popular Cults (End of 2nd century B.C. and upto 3rd century A.D.)*

Inspired by the Buddhist monks, their zeal and monastic order the traders had expanded their horizons a lot more. At Dharaṇikoṭa (Amarāvatī) and Kaveripattinam on the east coast wharfs with navigational channels have been found in levels datable to 2nd century B.C. Arikamedu (Poduke) has been a great Roman trading centre, precious objects apart, the rouletted ware (mostly large dishes, platters and bowls) appear in large numbers. Tāmralipti, Salihundam, Dharaṇikota, Arikamedu, Kaveripattinam, Uraiyur, Korkai and recently Alagankulam (Nagaswamy 1991) etc. have clearly shown that this pottery has an earlier horizon, say late 2nd century B.C. and indigenously manufactured as well. This ware is found with the Buddhist monasteries on the Bengal-Āndhra Coast. The imported Rouletted Ware along with Roman gold coins and precious objects, besides Arretine (Italy 25-50 A.D.) and Amphorae wares was greatly favoured by Indian merchants and Buddhists as well. So we find these three wares in good number in the early historical sites of India throughout, besides Śrī Lanka. (Anuradhapura, Kantarodai and Mantai, etc.) So far we have no evidence of these pottery wares from South-East Asian countries, like Thailand, Indonesia and Malaya, though a few Rouletted ware sherds were recently found from Coastal Java, and Bali. It may be seen that Buddhism and allied art objects occur in these Islands in later periods (Sarma, 1985) (5th century A.D. onwards) when compared to Śrī Lankan evidences. Nevertheless B.N. Mukherjee has made certain unique discoveries from the sites on Bengal Coast (Mukerjee 1989). He recognised, for the first time, numerous Kharoshṭī Bhāhmī inscriptions on pots, plaques and terracotta seals, from Chandraketugarh, Bengarh, Hadipur, Ataghara and Deulpos in district 24-Paraganas and Tamralipti Museum, Tamluk. Not only on the Bengal Coast but these Kharoshṭī-Brāhmī records on pottery and baked terracotta objects (circular seals and sealings) are now reported from Thailand and Bali too. It appears then that tradesmen coming from North-West (Gandhara and Oxus regions) moved through inland Mathura region to lower Gaṅgā-Yamuna doab and Madhyadēśa, reached the lower Gangetic Valley of Bengal (Bajpai 1989) in good numbers and then took to maritime routes to reach the South Asian countries. They mixed up with the local Brāhmī using merchants, who were Buddhists too and developed a mixed "Kharoshṭī-Brāhmī" writing with north-western *prākritic* expressions.Various types of sea-going vessels are depicted on the these terracotta seals and pottery vases (corn, horses and soldiers). Uninscribed copper cast coins from Harinarayanapur near the estuary of Ganges possessed rare designs of ship. The terracotta sealings found at Chandraketugarh bear impressions of full rigged ships.

These objects, like the Roman wares noted above, end up by 3rd century A.D. It appears to be necessary to plan for a more careful research followed by archaeological excavations in the sea-locked lands of South-East Asia, to find out, whether any Roman pottery wares and object of exchanges in early historical contexts are available. The pottery seals and sealings with Kharoshṭī-Brāhmī legends and ships on them reported from Thailand-Bali areas are of utmost importance in this regard.

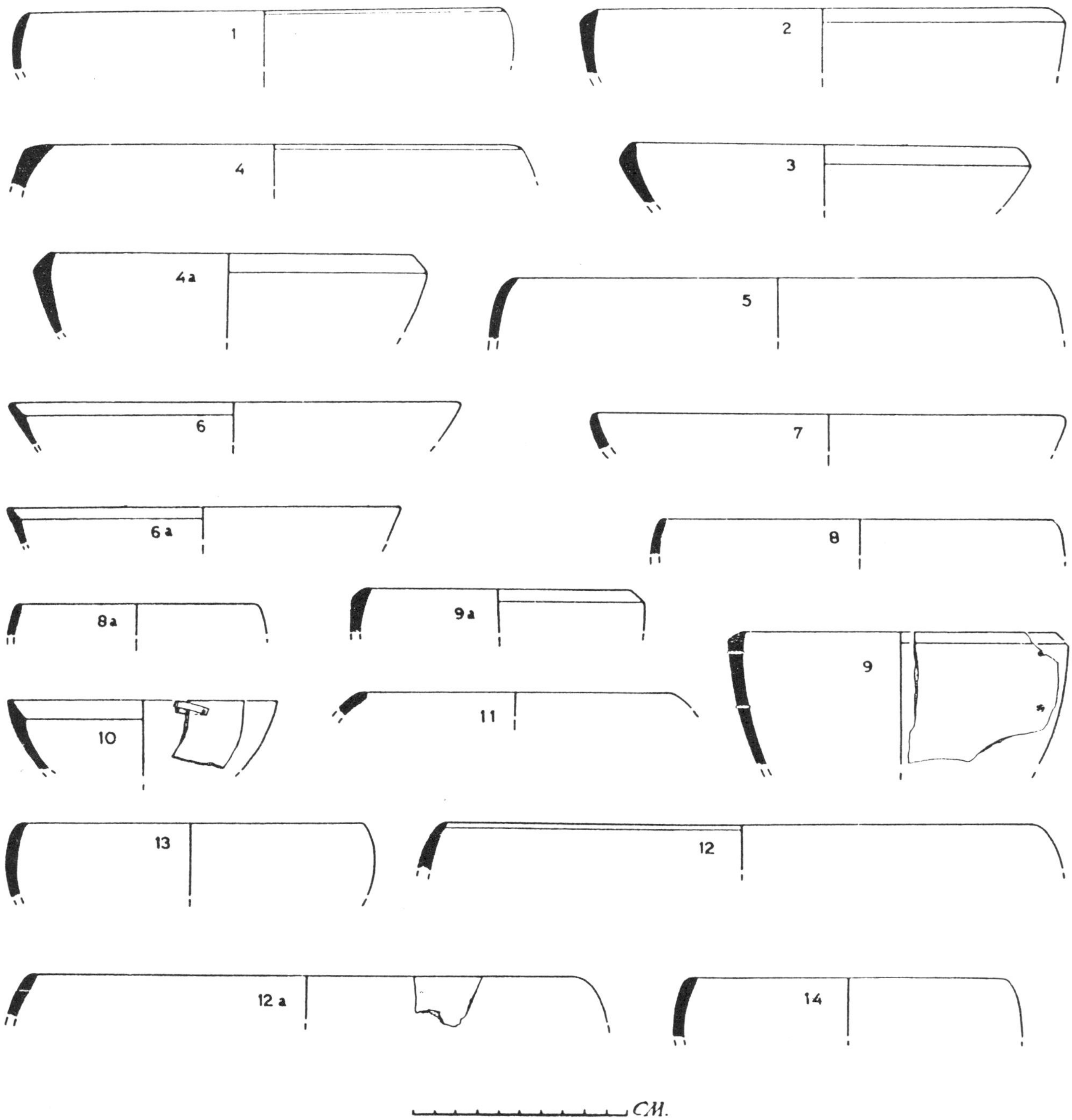

Fig. 2 : Amaravati, NBP Ware, Bowls and Dishes; Mauryan Phase (I A)

III. *Later Historical Periods: Post Buddhist and Medieval (circa, 9th to 17th century A.D.):*

This period is characterised by more influences from Far East and South China. The prolific Chinese Ceramics paved their way to the various port towns of South-East Asian countries- Phillippines, Indonesia, Malayasia, Thailand, besides India which had manifold trade relations. As we shall see the ceramics are mostly associated with the forts and palaces - less within Hindu temples and mosques during this long period. Commerce overtook culture.

There appears to be two distinct waves. The earlier dated to 9th-13th century A.D. and the second from - 14th to 17th century A.D. The former consisted of a few whitish porcelain confined largely to the coastal tracts of Āndhra and Tamilnadu. Noboru Karashima of Tokyo University along with some Indian colleagues (Madras and Calicut Universities) has been doing extensive field work on the Chinese potteies, their distributional patterns. etc. (Karashima 1989). More frequently the Chinese ships touched the South-East Indian ports during the Chōḷa times. From Gangaikondacholapuram and Darasuram digs, white porcelaiin was reported. It is well known that Chola emperors Rājā Rājā(I) and Rājendra sent various embassies to China. Even brāhmaṇical temples were raised and patronised in South China (Ray 1989) Chinese porcelain finds attributed to the Jindezhen kilns were found from Periyapattinam, Palaya-Kaya, Devipattinam and Nagapattinam which add substantially to our knowledge on the subject (Karashima 1990).

The site, Khalkatpatna, District Puri, Orissa located about 11 km. east of the Sun Temple, Konarak on the left bank of the River Kushabhadra, and 3 km. south-west of the sea-coast was excavated by the Archaeological Survey of India in recent years.

The discovery of one complete (PL. 3). and two fragmentary Chinese copper coins with square perforation in the centre bearing legend in Chinese characters on both obverse and reverse, Celadon Ware, egg-white glazed and glazed chocolate wares of Arabian origin suggest that Khalkatpatna served as a port-town during *circa* twelth-fourteenth century A.D., having maritime trade both with the countries of the west as well as east.

Soon after Chōḷas, the Kākatīyas of Warangal rejuvenated the sea-borne foreign trade. (Sarma 1990). Marcopolo visited the port of Mottupalli, called *Dēśūyakkoṇḍa Paṭṭana,* located in Chirala taluk, district Prakasam of A.P. I venture to identify this great port town with *Dabadan* mentioned in the Daoyi Zhilue, an important 14th century Chinse work, although Karashima recently put forth the view that *Dabadan* is *Periya paṭṭinam, Periya (Da)* and *(badan)= paṭṭinam,* on linguistic grounds. The famous Mottupalli pillar inscription of Gaṇapatideva (A.D. 1244), is of far reaching importance as this edict assures safety to traders *(abhaya, Śasana)* arriving from all continents *(Svadeśi* and *Paradeśis)* risking the sea-voyage and its hazards like storm attacks and shipwrecks. The levies (usually 1:30) on the items of import and export have also been listed with great detail and speak of the flourishing international trade from this important seaport which was provided with ware houses. Besides, the mention of several continents, islands, foreign countries and cities specific mention of *Chīni* (China) is noteworthy. Confirming this epigraphical evidence is the Telugu work *Harivilāsamu* written by the poet Śrīnātha, (circa, 15h century) which details the trading countries in the Andhra Coast and the objects of import, particularly silks and pottery wares from China. The Vijayanagara kings, specially of Sangama family, had regular trade and culture contact with the Ming dynasty of China. Chinese annals record that Bukka I (A.D. 1357-1377) had sent an embassy to China in 1374 A.D. Among a variety of Chinese Porcelain wares, a perforated coin of Ming Young Lo (1402-1428), contemporary of Hari Hara-(1377-1404) is a noteworthy find from the Royal enclosure. The Chinse Deluxe ware with exquisite Blue, gold and green hues and scenes of mythical animals, architectural landscapes of Chinese port towns, bearing auspicious words in Chinese characters reveal the impact of such exchanges. A large number of dishes and vessels depict the scenes of Chinese port towns, architecture, ships approaching the coast (particularly from Gingee and Vellore forts of the Nāyaka rulers). The inscribed and painted Chinese porcelain and glazed pottery wares were encountered in the medieval fortified towns of Daultabad (Maharashtra) Golconda (A.P.), Bidar (Bahmani kings 1422-1436 A.D.) and Bijapur (Adil Shahis 1489-1686), in Karnataka, Champaner in Gujarat, Fatehpur Sikri and Purana Qila, Delhi. These bear the marks of Long Quan and Fujian kilns of 13-14th century A.D. The highly prized table wares from the *Jingdezhan kilns,* blue and white glazed or enamelled ones (Golkonda, Purana Qila and Red Fort examples) were popular among the Muslim rule. In the year 1988-89 Noboru Karashima surveyed some places on the Malabar coast between Kannanur, north of Calicut to Vilinjam, South of Trivendrum. Chinese wares and tiles were noted in the churches and mosques in Cochin, Kollam (Quilon) Kodungallur, etc. datable to 15th-17th century A.D.

Cenramics are not perishable as other objects of trade like spices, silks and other metal objects. They are available in good quantities and survive for longer duration in different climates. So ceramics are of special significance for the study of ancient maritime routes and cultural contacts between nations involved in coastal trade. More specially, the Chinese ceramics are a class by themselves fairly reliable in dating, depict a variety of scenses on them throwing light on the culture and life patterns of medieval China. These ceramics serve as authentic archival sources not only for the study of the Chinese cultural and commercial history but of great chronological value and help to cross-check the Indian evidences.

REFERENCES

Bajpai, Shiv G. 1989. Mathura, Trade Routes, Commerce and Communication Patterns from the Post Mauryan period to the end of Kushana Periods in Doris Srinivasan (Ed.), *Mathura The Cultural Heritage.* Varanasi: 45-58

Deraniyagala, S.U. 1989. Excavations in the Citadel of Anuradhapura - Gedige, A Preliminary Report in *Ancient Ceylon.* 6: 39-48

Gurumurthy S. 1981. *Ceramic Traditions of South India.* Madras: 122.

Sarma, I.K. 1990. Ancient Andhra Ports, Religious Centres and Sea. Faring in S.R. Rao (Ed.) *Marine Archaeology.* I Goa: 19-23.

Sarma, I.K. 1989. Northern Black Polished Ware from Amaravati Excavations in L.K. Tripathi (Ed.) *Prof. R.C. Majumdar Commemoration Volume. Bharati.* Banaras.

Karashima Noboru. 1989. Trade Relations between Tamilnadu and China during 13th-14th century A.D. in *Journal of East-West Maritime Relations.* Tokyo I.

Karashima Noboru. 1990. Discoveries of Chinese Ceramic Sherds on the Coasts of South India. Paper read at the *International Seminar UNESCO* Madras

Mukherjee, B.N. 1986. Decipherment of the Kharoshti-Brahmi Scripts, *Asiatic Society Monthly Bulletin,* XVIII. 8 Calcutta: 4-6, 9-10

Ray, Hari Prasad. 1989. Indian Settlements in Medieval China A Preliminary study. *Indian Journal of Asian Studies.* 1: 69-81.

Identification of Setavyā, the Ancient City of Kosala with Siswania and its Terracotta Art

B.R. MANI*

Siswania, lat. 26° 45′N and long. 82° 46′E is the name of a site having a series of mounds on the left bank of Kuwano or Kuwana river, a tributary of river Sarayu, in the Basti district of Uttar Pradesh. The site extends from Pachisa (Tāḍījot-Pachīsā) village towards its north upto Deoraon village towards north-west and the Śiva temple of Bhadesarnath (Bhadreśvaranātha) is also situated closeby where the Kuwano river takes a northerly course. The distance of Siswania from the District Court of Basti is about 6 kilometres in the south-easterly direction and the site is located close to the Basti-Mahuli road towards its south-west. From village Dharmupur near this road or from Sonupar a little ahead on the road the site situated within one kilometre can be approached through and admist country joining groves and fields.

The site was explored by Durgavati Tripathi and C. Mani in 1944. In course of explorations nearly two thousand ancient coins comprising punch marked, uninscribed copper cast, local and Ayodhya varieties, Indo-Greek and Kushan issues were collected. A large number of semi-precious stone beads, copper objects, glass beads and bangles, terracotta human and animal figurines, terracotta toy-carts, pestles, stamps and other objects were found. The discovery of a multi-socket terracotta coin-mould made the explorer C. Mani believe that the site represented a Maurya-Śuṅga wharf town.

In 1950, Mrs Tripathi presented a fine Śuṅga terracotta female plaque to the State Museum, Lucknow (Tripathi 1967). Mrs Tripathi wrote articles in 'Dharmadūta' (Mahabodhi Society, Sarnath) and 'Madhyama Mārga' (Buddha Vihara, Lucknow) identifying the Nagaraka nigama, Sundarikā river and Sundarika Bhāradwāja's hermitage on it referred to in the Pali Buddhist texts. She has identified the Sundarikā with the modern Kuwano (Tripathi 1966).

The site extending between Deoraon and Siswania and Dharmupur and Deoraon-Siswania was revisited by the author during 1975 and 1978. It was observed that the main site has an average height of above 20 metres. But as a whole the Deoraon-Siswania-Pachisa area makes a single archaeo-cultural complex alongwith the mounds on the river. The antiquarian remains in forms of Northern Black polished Ware and other associated ceramics were noticed at Dharmupur, but perhaps the site there might have been levelled earlier for cultivation.

Two clay sealings of C. 3rd-2nd century B.C. with legends 'Dhamalatasa' (Dharmalātasya) and 'Idadevasa' (Indradevasya), the former stamped with swastika symbol and the latter having ujjain symbol on it have been pubished by the author (1982).

There is no doubt that the site represents a large city of the pre-Christian era. As compared to Saheth-Maheth or Śrāvasti, the capital of Kosala in Buddha's time, representing the city site of Maheth and the monastic site of Jetavana as Saheth, the present complex has also two parts. the larger Siswania-Pachisa representing the city-site and the smaller Deoraon representing the monastic establishment. This is evident also from the etymological derivation of the

* Archaeological Survey of India, Delhi Circle, Safdarjung Tomb, New Delhi.

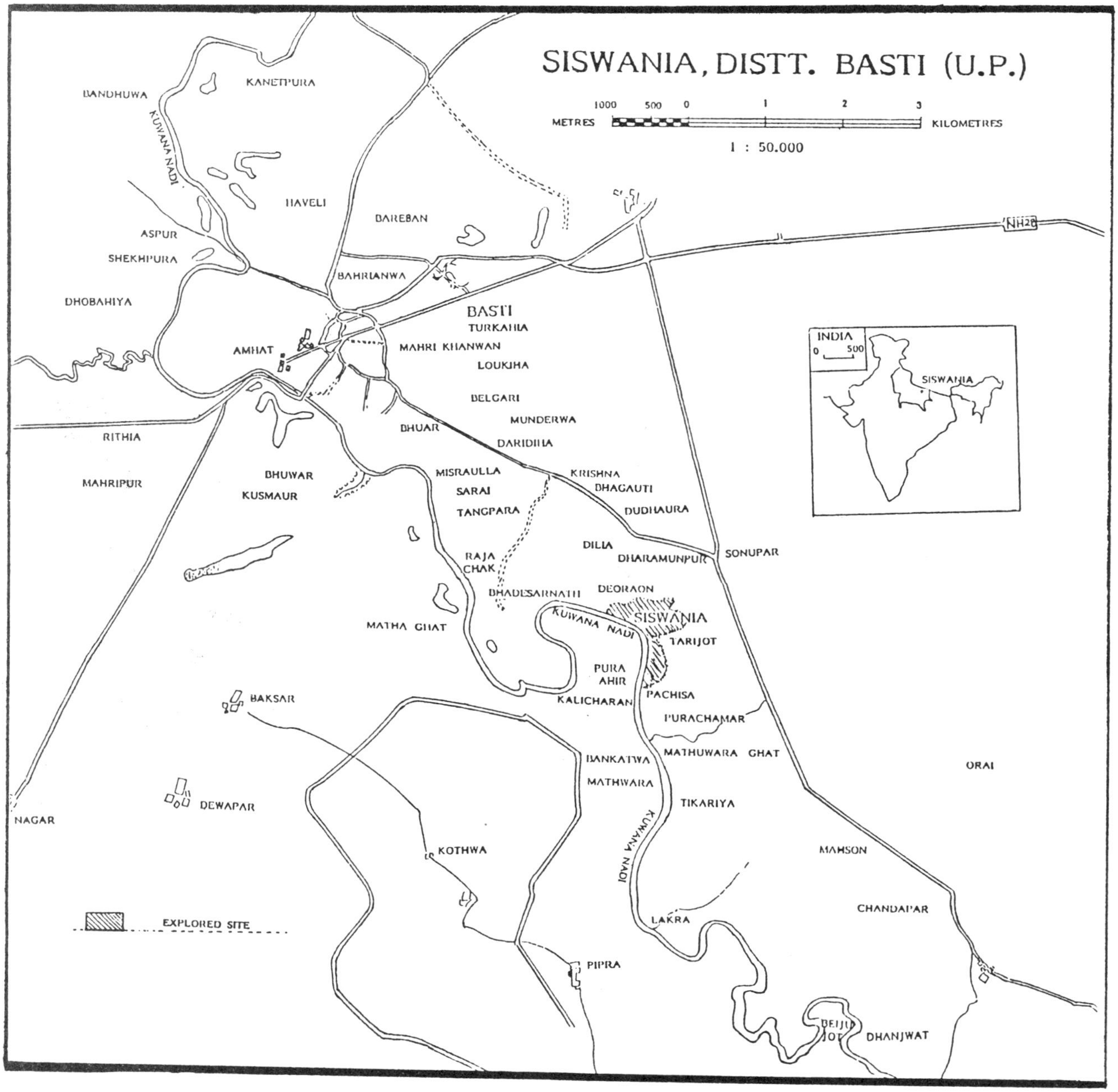
SISWANIA, DISTT. BASTI (U.P.)
1000 500 0 1 2 3
METRES KILOMETRES
1 : 50.000
INDIA
0 500
SISWANIA
NH28
BANDHUWA
KANETPURA
KUWANA NADI
HAVELI
BAREBAN
ASPUR
SHEKHPURA
BAHRIANWA
DHOBAHIYA
BASTI
TURKAHIA
AMHAT
MAHRI KHANWAN
LOUKJHA
BELGARI
MUNDERWA
RITHIA
BHUAR
DARIDIHA
MAHRIPUR
BHUWAR
KUSMAUR
MISRAULLA
SARAI
TANGPARA
KRISHNA
BHAGAUTI
DUDHAURA
DILIA
DHARAMUNPUR
SONUPAR
RAJA
CHAK
BHADESARNATH
DEORAON
SISWANIA
KUWANA NADI
TARIJOT
MATHA GHAT
PURA
AHIR
KALICHARAN
PACHISA
BAKSAR
PURACHAMAR
BANKATWA
MATHUWARA GHAT
MATHWARA
ORAI
TIKARIYA
DEWAPAR
NAGAR
KOTHWA
MAHSON
CHANDAPAR
EXPLORED SITE
LAKRA
PIPRA
DHANJWAT

name from Devārāma. The river Kuwano also played an important role in the urban development of the city-site, particularly, in transportation of merchandise and till recently mercantile barges were of common sight on this river.

The cultivation on the site has resulted in large scale levelling of the area. During the explorations of 1975 and 1978, ashy pits adjoining some burnt portions of earth looking like furnaces and large green patinated sheets of copper were noticed at the northern slope of the main mound where Rāma-Jānakī temple is in existence on the top of it. The vertical natural section towards the river showed a number of cultural assemblage and also evidence of large scale burning in one of the upper layers. The river too has cut a portion of the mound during floods in the past. The approximate maximum length of the site is about 1500 meters in north-west to south-east direction and about 600 metres width at the maximum.

A variety of shapes of pottery common in the area has been found at site; it comprised of grey ware, fine red ware, red slipped ware, chocolate slipped ware, black and red ware, black slipped ware, coarse red ware, Northern Black Polished Ware with sprinklers and other shapes in red polished ware.

Identification of Setavyā

The Nagaraka nigama of the Buddha's time was very positively across the river beside Chando tal at the place called Nagara. The village Pokhanni (Pushkariṇī) is located near Chando and was the seat of royal power till the Revolt of 1857. According to the *Sundarikabhāradvājasutta* the Buddha is said to have stayed among the people of Kosala on the bank of the river Sundarikā and had discussions with the Brāhmaṇa Sundarika-Bhāradvāja who resided there. The place seems to be Mahason or Mahāśrama on the left bank of kuwano and about 4 kilometres from Siswania on Basti-Mahuli road. Opposite Mahason and on the other side of the road is village Orai from where some excellent Kushan terracottas were found in the past by the explorer.

The famous *Pāyāsisutta* of the *Dīghanikāya* tells about the discourse by Kumāra Kassapa to Pāyāsi, the Brāhmaṇa chieftain of Setavyā on rebirth and Karma. In the introductory paragraph it has been said that Kumāra Kassapa who was once touring on foot in Kosala together with 500 monks stayed at Setavyā which was a city under Kosala. And there the venerable Kumāra Kassapa dwelt to the north of Setavyā town in *Siṃsapavana* or the grove of Śiṃśapā tree *(Dalbergia sisu)*.

The word *Pāyāsi* seems to have left its trail in village Pachisā where Pāyāsi resided in the southern part of the city and since his palace was located there the village which flourished was named after it. Siswania can be identified with *Siṃsapavana* which is still located towards north of Pachisa. Perhaps the place in the *Siṃsapavana* where Kumāra Kassapa stayed and preached *Pāyāsisutta* is represented by Deoraon (Devārāma) where in the following years monastery (ārāma) was established. Setavyā has been described as a place teeming with life, with much grassland and wood-land and with water and corn. King Pasenadi (Prasenajit) of Kosala had granted to Pāyāsi the domain as a royal gift with power to rule over it as if he was the king.

The Sutta adds: 'Then the Brahmins and house-holders of Setavyā, coming out from the town in companies and bands from each district so that they could be counted, went by the north gate, to the Simsapā-tree Grove'. They wanted to discuss and exchange views with Kumāra Kassapa and Pāyāsi has been described to have wondered about people going towards siṃsapavana when he observed them from the upper terrace of his house. After having been informed about the news by his doorkeeper, he sent words to them to wait for him for paying a visit to the wandering lord . Later he discussed with him in the company of brāhmaṇas and house holders.

In a passage in the Aṅguttara-Nikāya it is told that on a certain occasion when Buddha, 'the Exalted One was journeying along the highroad between Ukkaṭṭhā and Setabbya', the Brāhmaṇa Doṇa (Droṇa) who was also journeying along the highroad (addhānamagga) approached him and discussed. The highroad between Ukkaṭṭhā and Setavyā seems to be quite different from the highroad connecting setavyā with Śrāvastī on one hand and Kapilavastu or Kuśīnagara on the other. The exact identification of Ukkaṭṭhā is not yet certain, but under the circum-stances it might appear south-east of Siswania along-with the road leading to Mahuli. Ukkaṭṭhā has also been described in a Jātaka story to be connected with Vesāli and the Pali texts also refer to it in the vicinity of Ichānaṅgala-vanasaṇḍa and Subhagavana, constructed within an auspicious time with torches (ukkā) having been used at night. It had been donated as *brahmadeyya* by the king of kosala to Pokkharasāti (Sarao 1990).

The *Vatthugāthā* of the *Pārāyaṇavagga* of *Sutta-Nipāta* gives the important clue about the location of Setavyā in the context of the story of Bāvarī when he despatched a group of sixteen brāhmanas to get answers to some metaphysical questions from Buddha. They went from a place near Assaka beside Godavari river in the Deccan to Śrāvastī and thence to Rājagṛha to meet Buddha. They went from Śrāvastī (Sāvatthī) to Setavyā and Kapilavastu (Kapilavatthu) and then passed through Kuśīnagara (Kusinārā) town and Pāvā towards Vaiśālī (Vesāli) and to the capital of Magadha-

"Bāvariṁ abhivādetvā Katvā Ca naṁ padakkhiṇaṁ jaṭājinadharā sabbe pakkāmuṁ uttarāmukhā, Muḷakassa Patiṭṭhānam purimaṁ Māhissatiṁ tadā Ujjeniñ Cāpi Gonaddhaṁ Veḍisaṁ Vanasavhayaṁ. Kosambiṁ Cāpi Sāketaṁ Sāvatthiñ Ca Puruttamaṁ Setavyaṁ Kapilavatthuṁ Kusinārāñ ca mandiraṁ. Pāvañ ca bhoganagaraṁ Vesāliṁ Māgadhaṁ puraṁ Pāsāṇakañ cetiyañ ca ramaṇīyaṁ manoramaṁ"· (1010 to 1014).

This shows that Setavyā was located on one of the then most important highways which was frequented by the Buddha himself. This again confirms that Setavyā cannot be located towards west of Śrāvastī and it must be Siswania, the place having been mentioned as *Siṃsapavana* in the context of Setavyā in the *Dīghanikāya.*

W. Vost while identifying setavyā with *To-wai* of the Chinese travellers Fa-hian and Yuan Chwang Says 'The Chinese pilgrims tell us that a *Stūpa* was erected over the "relics of the entire body" of Kāśyapa Buddha at a place which Fa-hian names To-Wai, and located 50 *li to the west* or according to Yuan Chwang, who does not name the town, at a distance of 16 *li* (the *Life* gives 60 *li)* to the *north-west,* of Śrāvastī city. Both pilgrims, therefore, agree in placing the *Stūpa* of Kāśyapa Buddha to the *westward* of Śrāvastī city' (vost 1903).

The statement of two Chinese travellers regarding distance of the place from Śrāvastī are thus quite contrary. Vost further writes - 'To-Wai is, without a doubt, Setavyānagara, as the circumstance of the enshrining of an unbroken skeleton is "not related concerning any other Buddha" (Hardy, Manual, p. 88) except Kāśyapa. (The correct spelling should probably be kaśyapa, with the first a short.) The *Buddhavaṁśa* affirms that the Kaśyapa stūpa was located in the Sētavyāno garden in Sētavyānagaram (J.A.S. Bengal, Vol. VII, 1838, p. 797), and adds that the bones of this saint did not become disjointed even after cremation. It is remarkable that the identification of *To-Wai* with Setavyā has eluded the notice of the various translators of the itineraries of the pilgrims, and of scholars who have sifted the pilgrim's accounts for the rich store of geographical information available. For the reasons given I disagree with Mr. Vincent Smith's suggestion *(Remains near Kasia,* p. 4, note 3) that Setavyā will probably prove to be Sāhet Māhet.'

Vost's all arguments in favour of Setavyā as To-Wai are flimsy. Still believing To-Wai as Setavyā, on one hand but contrary to the Chinese accounts, he places Setavyā towards east of Śrāvastī on the basis of Pali suttas. His identification of Setavyā with Bāseḍilā (about 27° 24' N and 82° 20'E), a site six miles east from Balrampur and seventeen miles from Saheth Maheth is based on no cogent ground. His observation that the site is a large one and has yielded plain and moulded bricks, Kushan copper coins, a few terracotta objects and is surrounded by a number of tanks except in the north does not prove that the site is Setavyā. Moreover, on hearsay, he has tried to put that Burmese travellers visit the place and that he was informed that at Palṭīpur, about six miles to the south of Balrampur, some workmen chanced to encounter in an underground brick chamber a skeleton of a very tall man, which crumbled to dust on exposure to air. These seem to be mere concocted stories with no worth. The distance of Bāseḍilā from Śrāvastī seems to be very less in comparison with other cities mentioned in the context of Bāvarī in Sutta Nipāta and Siswania seems to be the better choice with a location at sufficient distance from Śrāvastī, Kapilvastu and Kuśīnagara on the main highway of the time.

Terracotta Art

Altogether there are 108 unpublished terracotta objects available at present for study. They are akin to the terracottas found from most of the contemporary Gangetic Valley sites.

They can be grouped as under:

(a) Human figurines	83
(b) Animal figurines	14
(c) Toy-Carts and rattle	3
(d) Utilitarian objects	8
Total	108

From the consensus of the terracottas from other sites of Gaṅgā Valley the human terracotta figurines of Siswania can be grouped into two broad chronological compartments. It is not possible to date them with accuracy in the absence of excavation. The first group is represented by archaic handmade figurines datable from about 6th Century B.C. to about 2nd Century A.D. and the moulded plaques mostly depicting female figures and belonging to Maurya-Śuṅga period (3rd Century B.C. to Ist Century B.C.). The second group is represented by handmade as well as moulded human heads some of which have foreign ethnic features and ritualistic figurines and heads with tenons below.

Among the archaic crude terracottas (Pl. XV), eight types continued from Pre-Maurya times to the first two centuries of the Christian era. Among these there are three handmade flat figurines, three distinct female figurines and a head. They have extended arms and pinched bird-like face and one of the female figurines and the head appear with fan shaped headgear with a hole in the centre, meant for hanging.

The female figurines have round and pointed breasts. There are two handmade figurines with pointed headress in the style of warrior figures dated to the beginning of the christian era with goat-like faces and slit mouths. They have necklace decorated in circles in bold relief. One of them with missing arms has broken legs and two incised circles that mark its breasts to be like the musician figurines as already reported from Piprahwa-Ganwaria and other sites. The other figurine, a bust of a male, holds two objects in its hands and splashes of red slip are still seen on it. The fourth type comprises four crudely finished and moulded female figurines (one represented only by a head) with broken arms and round breasts. They wear circular ear ornaments and a figurine of a baby is seen with these at the waist. The figurines possibly represent mother goddess. In a separate moulded type plaque the female figure is shown as in the previous type alongwith a baby but in this case the arms rest at the front side of the waist. The next type is represented by a hollow cylindrical headless torso of a female figure with a baby stuck near the left breast and two more crude figures below the baby, probably depicting two animals. In the next type there are two crudely made heads, with tenons below, one with bulging eyes wearing circular ear ornaments and the eyes made out of applique method and the other with slit mouth and pointed nose with two holes. The last type is represented by a handmade female figurine with pointed breast and extended arms. It is modelled in a sitting posture.

The profusely ornamented pieces are 3rd-2nd century B.C. terracotta plaques prepared with the help of a mould; they number 17. Among these the most interesting type is one represented by three female figurines with missing heads. They are shown wearing Sārī and ornaments like girdle, necklace and bracelets. The upper half of their bodies is bare and they are seen feeding some bird, possibly a parrot, with left hand holding some fruit below the breast and the right on the waist. Folds of the sārī are shown in the most beautiful and artistic fashion . Other broken plaques mostly represent female figures with head-dress of the time. The body proportions are quite realistic. Among these, the two broken terracotta plaques - the larger one found around 1950 and the smaller one by the author in 1975 with intact head portions are so similar that they seem to have been prepared by the same mould (Pl. XVI). The oval face with ear ornaments and well prepared hair style has the typical Śuṅga feature. They possibly hold a bundle of grass on their head. There are two plaques in which only the leg portions are extant and the figures are shown wearing anklets.

There is a small male bust wearing a round hat with knob on the top. The figure is slim but the hand and other parts of the body are missing. Similar terracottas have also been reported from Purana Qila excavations, New Delhi and are on display in the Purana-Qila site- museum, but are later in date. One more broken piece resembles it in style, colour and texture but wears a round cap.

An interesting handmade head with prominent incised eyes, eye-brows, pointed nose and slit mouth with prominent cheeck having a third eye on the forehead, depicted vertically may be identified with Śiva.

The remaining terracotta heads datable to the first two centuries of the Christian era can be classified into eleven sub-types as under-

1. Eleven comparatively larger terracotta heads, both moulded and handmade were executed in the sculptural style of the Kushan period. Interesting among them are: one with tenon below, and depicted with open mouth, circular ear ornament and horizontal hair locks (Pl. XVII); one female head with hair gathered and dressed in circular bun-style in front the common feature of Mathura art (Pl. XXI); three female crowned heads having an ornament stuck with forehead with a jewel in the middle giving a look of side-lock (Pls XXII-XXIV); a male head with moustaches shown with incised lines and bindī on the forehead with a tenon at the back side with incised circles showing the arrangement of hair (Pl. XVIII); a male head with moustaches and crown with circular jewel ornamentation (Pl XIX); a female head with crown giving a Hellenistic look and a male head with turban (Pl. XX).

2. Nine smaller terracotta heads with thick lips and large open eyes wearing fan shaped crowns, four of them wearing a jewel ornament on forehead, one of them having dotted ornamentation below the crown.

3. One flat handmade head with vertical incised lines showing the crown and pointed eyes, nose and lips.

4. Two female terracotta heads with fan shaped crown, open eyes and auspicious mark (bindī) on forehead.

5. Two male terracotta heads, one with moustaches and other with long lips having foreign ethnic features.

6. Six moulded and handmade terracotta heads with tenons below; one of them has an auspicious mark (bindī) on forehead.

7. Three moulded female terracotta heads wearing circular ear ornaments and headdress arranged alongwith crown, pointed nose with nostrils and dotted decoration on forehead alongwith eyebrows; tenons below.

8. One male terracotta head with typical Scytho-Kushan ethnic features executed in a refined manner with tenon below and wearing the ornament stuck on forehead and front sides looking like side-locks.

9. One female terracotta head with fan shaped crown and necklace, with round face, pointed nose, open mouth and round eyes.

10. Five terracotta heads, three moulded and two handmade. One of the moulded heads has a circular ornament on forehead.

11. One female handmade head with open mouth, large eyes, pointed nose having auspicious mark (bindī) on forehead and fanshaped crown with slanting bands.

There are two crudely modelled busts of female figurines - one with pointed breasts and wearing necklace and hair arranged in the shape of bun and the other with round breasts and wearing a peculiar elongated ear ornament. Both have auspicious mark (bindī) on their foreheads.

The most interesting Kushan female bust is a 16.5 cm. high terracotta figurine modelled from all the sides with prominent eyes, lips, pointed nose and pointed breasts. It wears a fan like headgear with incised marks, circular flower shaped ear ornaments, double necklace and an ornament on the upper part of the arm in the shape of *bhujabandha*. The hair is arranged in the back side in a single tress formation.

There are altogether fourteen animal figurines-two elephants, four horses and seven bulls besides one plaque showing a seated figure looking like a monkey with folded hands holding some indistinct object. The elephants are profusely decorated with incised lines and circular ornamentation. Three of the four horses are similarly decorated and applique bands are attached for ornamentation. Among the bulls, one has a vertical hole in the centre and horizontal hole in the back. Another bull has two types of stamped decoration - one with a circle divided into four compartments and each having a dot in relief and the other with herring-bone pattern.

Among the three toy carts and rattle, one is in standard shape with holes in front and back for fixing axle for wheels. One wheel of a toy cart has also been found. The third is a broken piece of rattle with holes passing from the front to the back and through the body for the axle for fixing two wheels. This is a bird-shaped piece with swollen body having stamped decorations of sun and dots on the upper surface of its body.

Among the utilitarian objects there is a mould with oval socket in the centre, three pestles, one rectangular skin rubber with straight lines, two stamps with circular design with radiating lines and an oblong piece with three holes in a line, whose functional purpose is not clear.

It has been shown in the first section that on the basis of Pali Buddhist texts and other facts now available the modern Siswania can be identified as the ancient Setavyā. Until the site is fully excavated, archaeologists have to remain satisfied with this identification.

Analysis and evolution of the terracottas in the context of social surroundings, clay and symbolic content alongwith ceramic production can be possible when the site is excavated and artifacts *(vas sacra and in other forms)* are considered in the light of associated finds of stratified deposits*.

* The inspiration for writing this article, I owe to my father, Shri C. Mani who has originally explored this site as far back as in 1944 with my grandmother Shrimati Durgavati Tripathi and uncle shri C.D. Tripathi, I.A.S. I am grateful to all the above savants of archaeology for bringing this site on the archaeological map of India.

REFERENCES

Dighanikaya, Pali Text Society, London. II. 316: 349-74 (3 volumes ed. by Rhys Davids, T.W. and Carpenter, J.E. 1890-1911 and 1957).

Mani, B.R. 1982. Some Seals, Sealings And Stamps In My Collection. *Journal of the Numismatic Society of India.* XLIV. Pl. VI. 8-9: 86-87.

Sarao, K.T.S. 1990. Urban Centres and Urbanisation As Reflected In the Pali Vinaya And Sutta Pitakas. Delhi: 118.

Spence Hardy, R. 1853. *A Manual of Buddhism* (reprinted Varanasi 1967): 86. At one place Spence Hardy also writes 'In the Amawatura, Buddha is said to have passed from Setawya to Kapila, and thence to Kusinara, in going from Sewet to Rajagaha (p. 133).

Sutta-Nipata, translated and edited by Lord Chalmers. 1932. London. Vagga 3, Sutta 4. 455-86: 106-144.

The Book of Gradual Sayings (Anguttara Nikaya), translated by Woodward, F.L. Bombay. 1933. Vol. II. VI (36):43.

Tripathi, Chandrabali. 1967. *Bharatiya Samaj men Nari Adarshon Ka Vikas* (Hindi). varanasi : 210-11; q.v. *Uttar Pradesh Ke Sangrahalayon Ki Unnati Tatha Karya Vivarana 1950. Lucknow: 40.*

Tripathi, Durgavati. 1966. Prachin Kosala Janapada Ka Nagaraka aur Uske Aitihasik Prasang (Hindi). *Dharmaduta,* March-April 1966, Sarnath 175-177.

Vost, W. 1903. Setavya Or To-Wai, *Journal of the Royal Asiatic Society:* 513-16.

Role of the Individual's Perception and Important Explanatory Modes in Archaeology

VIJNESHU MOHAN*

In India, archaeology is often criticized as being overwhelmingly descriptive. Barring a few exceptions, archaeology in India, seems to be mainly concerned with descriptions of the material remains of past human societies. Of late, however, advances are being made towards laying a greater exphasis on the related explanatory aspects of the growing discipline. Problem oriented researches are more frequently undertaken with the aim to integrate the theory data relationship, Also, coordinated research is gaining ascendancy in conjunction with allied scientific fields. With the relatively recent spur in theoretical literature, Indian archaeology too appears to be yearning to enter the mainstream of archaeological thought.

The present article seeks to review the most recent literature in the context of the role of explanation in archaeology on a global scale. There is apparently a general enthusiasm due to the "promise"rather than the "current products" of the so-called new archaeology (Fagan 1986: 210, Miller 1982: 94). The archaeological discipline is continually and rapidly evolving as more and more archaeologists become inclined to interact with the now available foundations of theory building or begin to "dig for ideas" (Carver 1989 666.74).

The role of individual perception and its bearing on the theory data relationship:

* 1293, Sector-13, Urban Estate, Kurukshetra.

How do we form ideas in an archaeological context? It is the ambience of an archaeologist that conditions the formation of ideas for understanding of the past material remains. The perception of the modern society gets inadvertently projected into the inferential framework abut the past (Allchin 1985: 21, Dhavalikar 1983: 49-68, Lyton 1984: 64-65, Orme 1981: 22-23, Zubrow 1980: 22).

The task of theory building is further complicated and constrained by the fact that archaeology can never be repeated (Renfrew 1983b: 7, Trigger 194: 292). Furthermore, it needs to be understood that theory and data are inseparable. Worthwhile theory building cannot proceed, albeit inductively, in the absence of an adequate data base. On the other hand, in the deductive mode of inferential progression it is the hypothesis that dictates the collection of data set. Both theory and data are, therefore, interactively linked in the process of archaeological explanation (Gardin 1980: 101-4).

It is another matter, however, that the judgmental level continues to significantly influence the archaeological thought. King states that "it is impossible to get all information in archaeology, this will seriously impair the usefulness of data even for eventual inductive synthesis" (King 1971: 261). Under this fairly well known adage, archaeologists must eschew rigidity in their stance for ultimate answers. The best option would be to properly relate theory to data option would be to properly relate theory to data (Hodder 1985: 11, Renfrew 1981: 258, Fleming and Johnson 1990: 306). Here, the importance of the data base is self-evident in the sense that descriptive data is no less essential for statisfactorily testing the hypothesis or building theories. But, it is appropriate to postulate that theories cannot be judged by other theories, thus, highlighting an urgency for verifiable observations (Reece 1987: 112).

By an Indian school of logic, among others, the theory data relationships are based on the intuitive inferences *(anumāna)* which are in turn based on reality *(darśana)* or its experience *(anubhava)* of individuals. Obviously, because of the element of intuition, the knowledge of the past is imperfect. This is duly envisaged in what is now known as the terminal sceptical crisis of the 1980s (Watson 1986: 450-51). As the ideological makeup of the archaeologists and that of the past dwellers may not coincide, the resulting explanations are bound to remain conjectural, unreal or counter-factual (Apel 1984: 4, Case 1973: 39). Therefore, it becomes essential to explore the ideational realm of the cultural components. The so-called archaeology of mind (Renfrew 1982 Leone 1982) is recently attempted with a renewed vigour. At the same time, however, it is considered to be inadequate for verifying statements about ideas in the prehistoric people's head and consequently the archaeologists are thought of as only building assumption upon assumption (Hodder 1984: 28). Actually, the mental constructs of the archaeologists also help to shape up the explanations. It is more important, therefore, that the researchers strive to be explicit about their goals, methods and techniques (Martin 1971: 6). The problem may even then continue to be unresolved because the preoccupation or bias with certain ideas is likely to yield distorted explanaitons. There is no denying that the present molds the study of the past. Latter's reconstruction is like a "social sentiment" in the present (Hodder 1985: 18). The similar view that inference, in general, springs from perception is subscribed to by the Indian school of philosophical thought, as early as, known by the nineteenth century studies (Bird 1840, Bodas 1897. Both the conscious and the subconscious level, the explanations in the archaeological context remain to be moderately speculative. Their adequacy could be judged in the light of the correlation between theory and data. A satisfactory level of explanation is more likely to be reached with the dilution of the debate between the "deep-diggers" and the sceptical "offsite" archaeologist A two way theory-data relationship naturally enhances the adequacy of archaeological explanations (Snodgrass 1985: 32).

The perceived box is proposed to replace Clarke's Black box whereby the former is dependent on the observer's view point (Clarke 1968, Hodder 1984: 27). The observer may be highly objective but an obsession with trying to bring out ultimate answers (see above) may turn out to be merely a wateful exercise or a *kākadanta-parīkṣā* (search for teetch in a crow), in the old Indian logical terms. The perception of researcher may not act as a catalyst to the flow of the theory data relationship. However, as in geographical sciences, simplification of complex issues facilitates progress. Besides attempting to simplify, the archaeologists should nevertheless be aware of the role of speculation in explanations. Often the missing information is not only retrieved but also formalized by speculations and conjectures. The proximity of speculations to the past reality is, at least, subconsciously conditioned or governed by the subjective perception of the contemporary society.

The usefulness of systems approach

The movement of the new archaeology began in the 50s and 60s of the present century. Culture is defined, by one of its exponents, as the extrasomatic means of adoptive system which is employed in the integration of society with its environment and socio-cultural subsystem (Binford 1968). The system is considered as non-passive and the inherent dynamic changes are regarded to be due to the interaction with the arbitrarily divided sub-systems of population, subsistence, technology, society, trade and projection. The inevitable changes take place with or without an external stimulus. In a homeostatic system the changfe is, thus, endogenous or from with the system.

The systems approach mainly deals with measurable variables. How do we then account for the past beliefs, meanings, etc.? Although a projective subsystem interacts within the system yet it apparently falls short of the explanation for the ideational realm. Even, the processual approach is deterministic! For example, in the processual view the invidual s are regarded as submerged with the systemic exigencies (Hodder 1985: 7-8).

Deductive logic in archaeological explanations

Nomological-deductive or hypothetico-deductive methods of explanations are those where the hypothetical observations or their negations employ a gradual testing of datas. In the nomological deductive approach law like generalizations are applied to observations or premises. Gregory has given a graphic representation of the two approaches as follows:

L_i-- L_r (Laws)		T_i--	(Theory)
C_i--C_n (Initial conditions)		H_i--H_i	(Hypotheses)
E-- (Event)		C_i--C_n	(Initial conditions)
		E'--	(Event)
		(After Gregory 1978: 34)	

These explanations may be criticized as being basically inductive like any other "covering law" explanations (Watson 1984: 7). It must again be emphasized, however, that the familiarity of the archaeologist or researcher with the data draws those theoretical objectives which lead to the structing principles. Thus:

Archaeologist	data
	theoretical objectives
	conceptual links
	structing principles.
	(after Shanks and Telley 1987: 112, also see Renfrew 1977: 91).

But, in a recent review article Krishtiansen, has aptly though cautiously argued that, in archaeology, as the observable is to be explained in terms of the unobservable relationships, therefore, the impending explanations cannot simply be reduced to cause and effect regularities. As a corollary we may state that the law like generalizations are difficult, if not impossible, to achieve in archaeology.

The hypothetical approach is, in fact, not new to archaeology. It was implicity applied in traditional archaeology. On the basis of Walter Taylor's conjunctive approach, Paddayya (1988-89: 239, 245) concludes that the hypothetical method was applied as early as the middle of this century.

To illustrate its usefulness, when, for example, archaeologists are faced with the observable evidence or data of a clay model of a plough from Banawali (Bisht 1987: 150), then it may be employed to conceive the site as an agro-based semi-urban centre. This hypothetical objective can be further extrapolated to structure the presence of a truncated urbanism in a regional context of the Harappan civilization.

Such explanations are liable to be conjectural or probabilistic and hence inductive in nature. But, generally speaking the attempts at applying mathematical or statistical methods have not met with much success, especially, in the Indian context. For example, we are told of the failure of the sampling techniques at Walki. It may suffice to state here that there is an "inadequate relationship between statics (archaeological residue) and dynamics (human behaviors) (Hodder 1985: 10-11, Bogucki 1985: 785, Hodder 1986: 3, Srivastava 1988: 48). As Jennings (1985: 28) would say, archaeological thought variously manifests itself as 'the pendulum of orthodoxy swings".

Looking back, search for historicity in archaeological explanations

It is fairly well-known that during the initial phases of the new archaeology, the chronological assumption was largely regarded as anathema (Dunnell 1985: 297). Recently, however, a renewed emphasis is justifiably laid upon the recognition of the chronological horizon. A series of events is proposed to be identified in an "aquatic metaphor" instead of the "billiard ball metaphor" of the systems approach (Hodder 1987: 1-2). Moving backwards, archaeology has seemingly enshrined the time tested and basic importance of the time dimension in ahistorical framework.

The limited applicability of the Marxist approach

Experiments are undertaken for the application of Marxist principle to the study of archaeological material remains. However, this approach is found to be useful only for the historicity of the archaeological findings and it fails to "provide a methodology for recovering and processing archaeological data" (Trigger 1983: 5) Nonetheless, explanations based on the Marxist materialism are quite common. The dialectical mechanisms can be shown to operate as:

Infrastructure/base/mode of production

Forces of production Means of production	Social relations of Production Organization of production

V_s

Super Structure

Judicial Political — Ideology

(after Hodder 1986: 59)

Sztomka's (1947: 71) systemic functional representation of the Marxist model is essentially the same as above. The classification of Childe's (for example 1950, 1958) explanations as Marxist is debatable. These explanations are not amenable to be treated as totally Marxist in approach. In the Indian archaeology the interpretations offered by Malik (1968, 1975) apper to be the closest to the Marxian model. The more recent Marxian approaches differ in that they emphasize the role of resources (for example Trigger 1984).

Symbolic interpretations as instruments of explanation

The findings of the symbolic archaeology seem to favour a historic mode of explanation and decry generalizations from one culture to another (Hodder 1986: 1-6). This symbolic approach is essentially ideographic or normative. It is evidenced in the utilization of contemporary language to translate the past texts (Hodder 1986: 178, also see the sections on the role of individual perception). An archaeologist must aspire to bring about a high level of objectivity in the explanations in orderr to minimize the influence of the ideographical dimension. Neeless to say, however, proximity to objectivity is attainable after the thorough knowledge of the available data. Sankalia has, therefore, besides many others rightly stressed the need for mastery over data prior to its interpretation (Sankalia 1979: 125).

The possibility of astrological predictions for archaeological explanations

A brief digression into an altogether different and perhaps "unscientific" methodology raises hopes for the development of astrological or astronomical archaeology (see, for example, Aveni 1980, 1984, Voiret 1987: 263). There is, at least, one attempt where astrology bears testimony to the antiquity of the Aryans in Indian (Ketkar 1904). In the more recent times, Sankalia has briefly hinted at the usefulness of the astrological prediction for the interpretation of the decay of the Indus Civilization (Sankalia 1989: 6). Admittedly, as astrology is an interpretative "science", the explanations thus based are found to be subjective due to the involvement of double assumptions.

Concluding remarks

Most of the archaeological explanations are, by their very nature,.no better than inferences *(anumāna)*. Only a rational response may lessen the confusion generated by the irrationality that permeates the explanations (see Feder 1984: 536). There is an urgency for the discovery of inventive thought. Not too infrequently, the criticism of the new archaeology as "a horrid example of scientism" seems justifiable (Gibbon 1984: 116). So much so, that the fear for what is allegorically termed as "pseudo-archaeology" (Fagan 1987: 2-3, also see Daniel 1981: 192) is not altogether unfounded.

The foregoing review highlights the various explanatory approaches in archaeology. The basic theme of concordance in theory and data runs through almost all the approaches. The viability of these explanatory modes of explanation is a matter of personal choice and training. This article is not meant to utterly undermine traditional describe archaeology. As already stated, detailed descriptions are conductive to the generation of theories. In fact, as Hodder would say (1989: 274) even older ideas could be safely worked in new ways.

BIBLIOGRAPHY

Allchin, B. 1985. Enthnoarchaeology in south Asia. In Schostmans, J. and M. Taddei (eds). *South Asian Archaeology 1983.* Naples, Institute Unversitario Orientale: 21-34.

Apel, K.O. 1984. *Understanding and Explanation.* Cambridge. The MIT Press (Warke, G.Translator).

Aveni, A.F. 1980. *Skywatchers of ancient Mexico.* Austin. University of Texas Press.

Binford, L.R. 1968. Archaeological perspectives. In Binford, L.R. and S. Binford (eds) *New Perspectives in archaeology*. Chicago. Aldine: 5: 32.

Bird, J. 1840. On the historical geography of Hindustan, and the origin of the social state among the Hindus. *Journal of the Asiatic Society of Bengal* 9/2: 848-58.

Bisht, R.S. 1987. Further excavation at Banawali 1983-84. In Pande, B.M. and B.D. Chattopadhyaya (eds.) *Archaeology and History*. Delhi. Agam Kala Prakashan. 135-56.

Bodas M.K. 1895-97. A historical survey of Indian logic. *The Journal of the Bombay Branch of the Royal Asiatic Society* 11: 306-47.

Bogucki, P. 1985. Theoretical directions in European archaeology. *American Antiquity*. 50: 780-88.

Carver, M. O.H. 1989. Digging for ideas. *Antiquity*. 63: 666-74.

Case, H. 1973. Illusion and meaning. In Renfrew, C. (ed.) *The explanation of culture change: models in prehistory*. London. Duckworth: 35-46.

Clarke, D.L. 1968. *Analytical Archaeology*. London. Methuen.

Daniel, G. 1981. *A short history of archaeology*. London, Thames and Hudson.

Dhavalikar, M.K. 1983. Ethnoarchaeology in Inida. *Bulletin of Deccan College Research Institute*. 42: 49-68.

Dunnel, R.C. 1985. Archaeological survey in the lower Mississippi alluvival valley 1940-7: a land-mark study in American archaeology. *American Antiquity*. 50: 297-301.

Fagan, B.M. 1986. American archaeology: past and future. *Antiquity*. 60: 210-3

Fagan, B.M. 1987. Archaeology and pseudo archaeology. *Expedition*. 60: 210-3

Feder, K.L. 1984. Irrationality and popular archaeology. *American Antiquity*. 49: 525-41.

Fleming, A. and M. Johnson. (eds.) 1990. The Theoretical archaeology Group (TAG).: origins, retrospect, prospect. *Antiquity*. 64: 303-6.

Gardin, J.Q. 1980. *Archaeological constructs*. Cambridge. Cambridge University Press.

Gibbon, G. 1984. *Anthropological archaeology*. New York. Columbia University Press.

Gupta, S.P. 1972-73. Model for first urbanization in India. *Puratatva*. 6: 42-4.

Hodder, I. 1984. Archaeology in 1984. *Antiquity*. 58: 25-32.

Hodder, I. 1985. Post processual archaeology. In Schifer, M.B. (ed.) *Advances in archaeological method and theory*. 8. Orlando. Academic Press: 1-26.

Hodder, I. 1986. *Reading the past*. Cambridge. Cambridge University Press.

Hodder, I. 1987. The contribution of the long term. In Hodder, I. (ed.) *Archaeology as long-term history*. Cambridge. Cambridge University Press. 1-8.

Hodder, I. 1989. Writing archaeology: site reports in context. *Antiquity*. 63: 268-74.

Jennings, J.D. 1985. River basin surveys: orgins, operations, and results, 1945-69. *American Antiquity*. 50: 281-96.

Ketkar, V.B. 1904. Astronomy in its bearing on the anttiquity of the Aryans. *The journal of the Bombay Branch of the Royal Asiatic Society*. 21: 24-33.

King, J.J. 1971. A conflict of values in American archaeology. *American Antiquity*. 63: 255-62.

Lyton, N. 1984. The use of enthnoarchaeology in terpreting south Asia protohistory. In Kinnedy, K.A.R. and G. Possehl. (eds) *Studies in archaeology and polaeoanthropology of south Asia*. New Delhi. Oxford. 63-72.

Malik, S.C. 1968 *Indian civilization: the formative period*. Simla, Indian Institute of Advanced Studies.

Martin, P.S. 1971. The revolution in archaeology. *American Antiquity*. 36: 1-8.

Miller, D. 1982. Explanation and social theory in archeological practice. In Renfrew, C., M.J. Rowlands and B.A. Segraces (eds.) *Theory and explanation in archaeology*. New York. academic Press: 83-96.

Orme, B. 1981. *Anthropology for archaeologists*. London. Duckworth.

Paddayya, K. 1988-89. The role of hypothesis and traditional archaeology. *Bulletin of the Deccan College Research Institute*. 47: 239-246.

Reece, R. 1987. Thinking about archaeology. In Clayton, P.A. (ed.) *University of London Institute of Archaeology golden Jubilee Bulletin*. 24: 191-204.

Renfrew, C. 1977. Space, time and polity. In Friedman, J. and M.J. Rowlands (eds.) *The evolution of Social System*. London.Duckworth: 0-109.

Renfrew, C. 1981. Space, time and man, *Transactions of Institute of British Geographers*. 6: 257-68.

Renfrew, C. 1982. *Towards an archaeology of mind* Cambridge. Cambridge University Press.

Renfrew, C. 1983. Geography, archaeology and environment. *The Geographical Journal*. 149: 316-23.

Sankalia, H.D. 1979. *Born for archaeology*. Delhi. B.R. Publishing Corporation.

Sankalia, H.D. 1989. *Earthquake and civilization*. In Handa, D. (ed.) *Ajayaśrī* Delhi. Sundeep: 3-8.

Snodgrass, A.M. 1985. The new archaeology and the classical archaeologist. *American Journal of Archaeology*. 89: 31-37.

Srivastava, K.M. 1988. *New horizons of Indian archaeology*. New Delhi. Books and Books.

Sztomka, P. 1974. *System and function toward a theory of society*. New York. Academic Press.

Trigger, B.G. 1983. If Chld were alive today? *Bulletin of the Institute of Archaeology*. London. 19: 1-20.

Vioret, J.P. 1987. Theodilite measurements and computation of megalihic astronomical alignments in ancient Chile. In Reed, D.W. (ed.) *Spirit of enterprise*. Berrkshire. Von Nostrand Reinhold: 263-265.

Watson, P.J. LeBlane, S.A. and C.L. Redman 1984. *Archaeological explanation*. New York. Columbia University Press.

Watson, P.J. 1986. Archaeological interpretation, 1985. In Meltzor, D.J., D.D. Folwer and J.A. Sabloff (eds.) *American archaeology past and future*. Washington. Smithsonian Institution Press: 439-57.

Zubrow, E.B.W. 1980. International treds in theoretical archaeology. *Norwegian Archaeologicala Review*. 13/1: 14-23.

The Lady of the Beasts or The Lord of the Beasts A Reappraisal

P.V. PATHAK*

The famous Paśupati seal has been one of the most significant finds of the Indus culture. Although, the seal title is more or less established, the nature of the deity at the centre has been debated. Earlier Sullivan (1964) had expressed views that the deity was the "Mistress of Beasts" stating that hunting was clearly an important activity in the peasant communities of Sind and Baluchistan. He concludes: ' It is not unlikely, then, that the goddess should have been not only the giver of vegetational life but also the "Mistress of beasts" and the patroness of the hunt.' He drew attention to two other seals where pigtails of the deity are clearly visible on seals. Latest addition to this controversy is an article by Atre (1985). According to Atre, the deity on the seal is neither the lord of beasts, nor the mother Goddess but is 'the virgin of beasts'. In support of her views, Atre has drawn parallels with the other seals representing the same deity and the mother Goddess statues from the Indus culture. She has also drawn parallels of a pictorial representation on the seal from Kalibangan with the Greek ritual of female sacrifice and concludes that the deity on the Paśupati seal represents the virgin of beasts, a female deity.

In the present article I have refuted the view of the central deity being a female deity by comparisons with the rituals and internal parallels supplied by other seals from the Indus culture. The methodology as recorded in ancient literature is more or less accepted in the field of the Indus culture studies.

* Surya Niketan, Mota Randha, Union Territory of Dadra, Nagar, Haveli.

Methodology

So long as a bilingual seal or graffiti is not traced or found the decipherment of the Indus seals will have to be attempted by comparison and parallels. Asko Parpola (1985) has given three widely accepted routes for drawing parallels and interpretation: 'There can be no doubt that three most important sources for interpretation are (1) the internal parallels supplied by the Harappan civilization itself, (2) the parallels offered by ancient West Asia, (3) those provided by the later civilizations. By later Indian civilizations Parpola implies the post-vedic period. But his contempt for those drawing parallels from the vedic civilization is not concealed, when he writes, 'while some fanatics especially in India have tried to force vedic analogies to back up their preconceived claims of the Aryan identity of the Indus people, the sobar scholars have usually cited parallels from the post vedic, classical Hinduism or from the modern times. These comparisons with Hinduism have often been accepted, at least tentatively, with the result that some identifications have been repeated from one book to another.' Here the personal bias of Paropola has overcome the true scholar within. Throughout the monograph, Parpola has drawn parallels from the vedic literature, however his sudden shift to the Dravidian roots is a different topic altogether. In support of his argument he repeats the theory propounded earlier, that the Aryans invaded the Indus region in two waves, first to come were Dāsas relatable to the Hissar III culture of the north eastern Iran and then came the Ṛgvedic Aryans. The Vedic literature is the outcome of these two successive large scale acculturations.

Atre too follows the same line of arguments. According to her, it will be more "appropriate that we free the Harappan civilization or to be more precise the Harappan religion from the narrow frame of either the vedic or of the later day Hindusism."

But it becomes equally difficult to accept the proposition to relate the so called virginity cult in the Indus civilization with the very late Diana worship in the Greek culture around 495 BC. It is as if the Indus culture and religion totally disappeared from the continental area extending from Afghanistan to Uttar Pradesh and from Himachal Pradesh to Diamabad in Maharashtra and took solid roots in the distant Greek islands after remaining dormant for centuries. On the other hand one finds such a smooth continuity of ideas from the Indus civilization, nay from the pre-Indus periods to the present day Hinduism that it becomes absolutely untenable to alienate the Indus religion and culture from the past and the present Hindu cultural ethos, inclusive of the vedic and the post-vedic periods.

If one is to follow Parpola regarding his views on drawing parallels from the classical and the present day Hinduism, obvious contradictions arise. If the Aryans had completely wiped out the Indus culture how could the post vedic and classical Hinduism be replete with the Indus culture antecedents, the Vedic culture remaining completely aloof. It was not so. There is continuity of cultural and religious belief ever since the pre Indus periods. Religious beliefs through symbols have been recurring since the pre-Indus period. Some of these are dealt with below. The list is not exhaustive, there are many more but only the prominent ones specially those referred to by Parpola are dealt with here.

Continuity of beiefs and reigious ideas

Aśvattha leaves and tree: Popularly known as pipal (Ficus religiosa) the tree has special singificance in the Vedic as well as later day Hindu religion. Its leaves were painted on the Indus pottery depicting sanctity. Parpola refers to the significane of the leaves in the Ṛgveda etc. The pipal tree appears to have acquired sanctity even before the Indus culture period. The pipal leaves are painted on the pottery of the Period IV at Mehergarh belonging to the third quarter of the 4th millennium and also on the Mundigak pottery belonging to the Period IV -1 of the immediate past of the Indus civilization time span. The pipal tree, branches and leaves are painted on several earthen pots of the Indus period. There are many Indus seals bearing the pipal leaf marks. In the vedic and post vedic and even the current Hindu tradition the Aśvattha occupies position akin to godhood. The analogy of Aśvattha in the Bhagadvad Gīta chapter XV chapter is famous.

Peacock: This bird is frequently painted on the pre-Indus culture pottery. Pottery at Mehergarh from the Period III belonging to the first half of the 4th millennium BC carries peacock designs (Jarrige 1977). There are innumerable such instances from the Indus culture which indicate that peacock had acquired not only aesthetic but also religious significance. Parpola states ' I would like to suggest that this bird, the peacock covered with many "eyes" or "stars" represents Varuṇa in his "sky garment" of the star spangled night.' In the Rgved it is above all Varuṇa who is watching from the sky with his eyes (sun, moon and the stars). The vedic funeral monument is built in the shape of a bird (cf. SB 13.8.3.9): it functions like the bird shaped fire altar with which Prajāpati flew up to the world of heaven (cf. SB 10.2.1.1) Parpola also gives the peacock figure from the Indus funerary pottery.

Swastika: Swastikas, both the right handed and left handed and also with decorations are painted on ancient Indian pottery. The Swastika pattern is painted on the pottery from Mehergarh since the pre-Indus period and from Mundigak (Casal 1961). There are several patterns of Swastika on the Indus pottery, seals and buttons, etc. Swastika is an unique symbol which though sacred has no folklore or legend associated with it. In the classical Hindu tradition which may be traced to a few centuries BC, Swastika stood as a sign for the Lord Gaṇeśa (Pandeya 1973). It may be said that the word 'Swasti' in the vedic literature meaning well being is represented by the symbol Swastika. The grid iron pattern of town planning of the Indus cities of Mohenjodaro and Harappa may appropriately be named after the Swastika pattern. As such, there is architectural pattern of house building named after Swastika. The symbol still occupies very prominent position in the Indian household. Ladies drawing Rangoli patterns for decoration start with drawing Swastika first. Thus in both the ritual and household tradition the Swastika symbol has occupied an unique position ever since the pre-Indus period.

Funeral rites: While in the near East the royal tombs dotted the land, no influence of the custom was observed in any of the Indus cemeteries, i.e. R 37 and H, etc. The bodies lay extended with head towards the north and legs to the south (Wheeler 1966) This is perfectly in tune with the age old belief of the south being the direction of the God of death, Yama. While the living human being is forbidden from sleeping directing legs to the south, the dead body is invariably laid with legs pointing to the south in India.

The custom of wearing bangles by ladies, adoring the Brāhmī bull, etc. still continue to be current in India ever since the pre-Indus period. There are many such beliefs and customs which appear to hold their sway ever since the pre-Indus period till to-date. How is it possible to isolate only the vedic, post-vedic or classical Hindusism from the religion of the Indus people? One regrets that an ace research scholar like Parpola deviates from the very obvious conclusions because of his bias for the so called Dravidian roots of the Indus culture. Similarly Atre's proposition of isolating the Indus culture from the ancient culture in India becomes irrelevant.

Mother or virgin

Atre points out that the mother goddess statues as found all over in the near Eastern and ancient Europen cultures are absent in the Indus culture. The typical nude female figurines with protruding breasts, heavy hips and belly portion, or where pregnancy seems to be the focal point of worship or sanctity are absent in the Indus culture. The female figurines of the Indus are not nude. On the contarry they are mostly the statues of shapely young maidens. Apparant contrast between the two types of the female statues can be easily verified from narly sixty illustrations presented by Agrawal. Of these the first 19 illustrations are of the typical mother Goddess type and found in the Western culture. From the illustration 20 onwards, the ancient female statues from the Indus and the neighbouring region are given (Agrawal 1984), while the mother goddess statues are least decorated, Atre rightly points out that the Indus female statues are invariably ornamented and clothed around waist and point to these being virgins. This trend also continues to the Pre-Indus times. The Mehergarh female statues of various periods as arranged by Jarrige also fit into the maiden - virgin pattern rather than the mother goddess pattern. As Atre points out, the statues serve some other purpose because, "the iconography of these figurines is not even in a single instance repeated on the seals and sealings which are equally important as a source of Harappan religion" (Atre 1986).

Were These the Playing Dolls?

It is also to be noted that though the female statues are of young, slim females, their features and ornaments are appallingly crude. Look at the artistic skills of the Indus artists, their expertise in carving numerous Indus seals with precision, the most proportionate statues from Harappa which can be envied by a modern sculptor, their skills in painting intricate patterns on excellently baked pottery and so also the impressionist mode of drawing animals on baked pottery; it is inconceivable that they could have fashioned the numerous female virgin statues in such a crude manner, if they were to be the object of adoration. But compare them with toys and toycarts, these are also equally unfinished and crude. The terracotta female statues and the animal toy figures from say Mundigak can be compared for this purpose. Although baked, they were not made very carefully, Wheeler too gives similar figures of terracotta bullock cart, the bulls, hen, dove, cat, etc. along with a figure of a beast looking like a boar covering his mouth with front legs. (Wheeler 1966). He further comments that the makers of terracotta at Mohenjodaro enjoyed a sense of humour, shown by numerous grotesque figurines. Thus these figures of the animals and maidens crudely made were toys for kids. While making these toys the artist did not pay much attention to make them attractive or aesthetically good looking. This trend was followed right till recent times, as late as early fifties and sixties. I remember the baked but crude toys which I used to play with, especially on the eve of Polā when oxen are worshipped annually on the new moon day of Śrāvṇa month of the Indian calendar. Many of these statues are half bust or made in sitting position on a broad base or pedestal. This is because the kid playing with them can position them easily. Piggot has given the figurines of women on broad bases from Kulli culture which have lavishly made hairdressing studded with ornaments. (Piggot 1961). The modern day kids in India are lucky to have not only the variety of toys made of different materials but they are aesthetically made with right features.

Populatin Trends

Considering the population trends, even during the Indus culture period, more than half of the human population must have been of youngsters below 15 years. There too the survival rate among the female children being higher, more than half the population of kids below 15 years must have been that of young girl - kids. Scholars and the Indus culture experts have overlooked this strata of society. Up to the age of 12 or so the kids needed some toys to play with. As it has been recalled till recent times, the female child preferred to play with dolls. And there are hardly any instance of the experts pointing to the female terracotta figurines being girls, toys especially made for them and not that they are less in number. The statistics of the female figurines is given by Marciar Fentres: "At Mohenjodaro a total of 136 figures were found, and at Harappa a total of 91, female figurines numbered 123 at Mohenjodaro and 69 at Harappa, confirming more or less to the expected 2 : 1 ratio. Male figures were in reverse proportion, 13 at Mohenjodaro and 22 at Harappa." (Marcia 1979). Fentress too states that there is no conclusive evidence that in the Indus culture human figurines functioned in a religious or ritual capacity. Nay they were dolls. One can understand that while the male child used to go out for playing outdoor games the girls used to play preferably indoor games, say dolls or *mock family affairs* imitating the female folk at home (known as Bhātukali in Marāṭhi) till recently say late fifties or sixties. They continued to play these indoor games till they attained the age of twelve. This trend must have been followed even during the Indus period so that apparently very large proporiton of female toys can be explained in the light of this social custom.

A question immediately arises as to why these toys were baked, and energy expended. The reason is also apparent. Since these toys and toy dolls were handled by kids mostly in the age group of say 3-8 years, those with calcium deficiency must have been inclined to suck those toys. Baked figures prevented the clay being sucked by kids. It was also appropriate that the dolls be of young females. Because the young girls must have been playing with them and therefore they were with hairdresses and ornaments. These statues must have inculcated in the minds of these girls that very soon they might have to prepare themselves like those female figurines and be married to suitable young men.

It can be concluded that the terracotta female figurines in the Indus civilization were neither mother goddesses nor the virgin goddesses but were toy dolls for young girls. They were the Indus culture maidens out to attract attention of young people enticing them with their attractive attire and lady's finger like shapely body. As Atre has rightly observed the figures of these statues are not to be seen on any of the Indus seals because they had no religious significance. They were mere toys.

The seal figures: male or female

In order to point to the feminine nature of the central figure on the Psśupati seal (No. 1) Atre points to a seal of cow woman and horned tiger from Mohenjodaro (Marshall 1232). The feminine character of the bending figure with horned headgear can be judged from the protruding breasts in half bent position.

Another characteristic of feminity of the central figure being the long plait of the central deity on similar Paśupati seal (Vats 1940) refers to a cylindrical seal from Kalibangan (Thapar 1979) which according to Atre, shows sacrifice of the virgin goddess.

Thus the above observations of Atre lead us to the following conclusion about the Indus civilization:

1. Female or female deity could be shown with horned headgear.

2. Long plait is indicative of female sex. i.e. it was only the female who used to maintain long hair as the Indian ladies do now. The corollary of this being that men did not maintain long hair but used to have their hair cut, or combed into a bun.

3a. Female figurines are clothed while male figurines are invaribly nude.

4. And as the Kalibangan seal depicts virgin sacrifice, there must have been the custom of virgin sacrifice prevalent in those times. All these conclusions are examined below.

Horned hedgear

Apart from the Paśupati seal referred to above, there is a triangular prism seal from Harappa referred by Paropala, where he has given the original three faces of the seal (after Vats 1940 Pl 93: 305) supplemented with rough sketches based on detailed autopsy copies drawn by him. In all these figures the human figure is wearing a horned headgear and it is shown to be ithyphallic in nature. Parpola compares these figures with proto-elamite seals from Susa where it is invariably the bull figures with similar headgear. Ithyplallic nature of the Paśupati seal will be dealt with in detail in the following sections.

There is already a seal of bull man from Mohenjodaro. As regards the cow woman seal, referred to by Atre the protruding breasts are obvious but the figure also appears to be phallic. Thus it is a composite figure, i.e. it has both the female type of breasts and also penis. It has headgear and a long tail. The original seal needs to be re-examined without any bias, as the seal photograph however enlarged does not help to come to very firm conclusion in this regard. If one were to go by bull man seal alone and Parpola's parallels with proto elaminite seals, this seal should be of a bull man rather than bull woman. But it is a very enigmatic figure.

Thus based on the triangular prism seal, the Paśupati seal and the comparison with proto elamite seals it can be concluded that horned headgear was shown only for male deity or figure and not for the female figure. Even in Western cave arts only the male figures were provided with pair of bovine or cervix horns (Leroi-Gourhan 1968).

There are two more observations that further support this conclusion. The demon Mahiṣāsura who was slain by Goddess Durgā is always shown with bovine horn headgear and he is male. When the tribal gonds of Madhya Pradesh, India, perform ritual dance wearing such horned headgears, it is always the male performer who wears it and not the female.

Long plaits

There are a) two male statues from Mohenjodaro with beard and bun and b) a statue of possible priest-king in sitting posture whose head is cut but the long curly hairs on the back can be clearly seen (Marshall 1931). And no single statue of a woman with long plait is available. But from the hair dressing they too appear to maintain long hair.

Thus it can be seen that long plaits are no sure indication of the figure being that of a female. It could also be a male figure.

Female sacrifice

According to Atre, the cylindrical seal from Kalibangan represents virgin sacrifice. This seal has two separate scenes. There are shown two human figures wearing bun and holding spear-like rod in their hands and a central figure with long plait. In addition there is one more composite figure of human torso and animal body. Of the three human figures the central figure is sacrificial victim, a virgin. This propostion raises certain doubts about the seal.

As already pointed out, the long plait is no sure indication of the figure being that of a female. But further inquires into sacrificial procedures point to the type of weapon to be used for killing a sacrificial victim. Normally the executioners prefer shorter weapons like dagger, axe, sickle, etc. in which case a strong single stroke severes the head of the sacrificial victim. This is to prevent him from being tortured before death.

Both the weapons held by human figures are curved spears with blades at one end. Thye are disproportionately long and being curved may not serve the purpose of killing instantaneously. Thus they are in no way useful for being used as weapons for sacrifice. There is a clear reference to the male sacrifice in the vedic lore in the story of Śunaḥśepa (Taittirīya Saṁhitā v.2.1.3) and Śatapatha Brāhmaṇa (XIII. 6). But the custom of female sacrifice is mentioned. On the contrary in the later Indian tradition the goddesses like Durgā, Kāli, were slayers of male demons.

It is not that virgin sacrifice was not at all prevalent in India. The virgins especially young girls before attaining puberty were sacrificed stealthily for acquiring wealth or lease of life for ailing person. But these were practised as black witch-craft and therefore never openly carried out with due sanction of soceity. Also such a victim was not offered in sacrifice to fire with due ceremony. While concluding her article, Atre states that 'addition of ploughshare and domestic fire which was regarded holy is sufficient to demonstrate the enhanced position of the primitive goddess. This position of modification and alteration at Kalibangan resulted in 'vestal fire' attaining the supreme importance as indicated by the presence of public as well as residential fire altars' (Atre 1986).

Thapar reports that at Kalibangan, no female figurines, neither cult objects depicting deity were found. Under these conditions, calling the fire altars at Kalibangan as 'vestal fire' and the proposition concluding the female-virgin sacrifice needs further re-examination And it will also have to be explained as to how the tradition of female sacrifice in vestal fire suddenly disappeared from India and took root in the Greek tradition after the lapse of nearly 1000 years or more.

Paśupati Seals

Terminology of Paśupati seal is applied to those Indus seals in which the central figure is sitting in folded legs position with both the hands stretched and wrists resting on the knees.

There are seven such seals reported so far.

Seal No. 1: Marshall Vol II PL XCIV - 420

Seal No. 2: Macay Vol II PL LXXVII - 222

Seal No. 3: Macay Vol II PL LXXVII-235

Seal No. 4: Masharll Vol III. PLC XVIII - VS 210

Seal No. 5: Marshall Vol III PLCXVI -29.

Seal NO. 6: Vats (1940) Vol II PLXCIII - 303.

Seal No. 7: Parpola (1979) has given a figure and reports it to be with the Ashmolean museum, Oxford.

In all these seals the central deity is seated in identical posture. Seal No. 5 is identical with seal No. 4 but engraving is much worn out. Excepting in seal No. 2 and 3, the central deity is surrounded by animals. Seal graffitti is clearly visible on seals Nos. 1,2,3 and partially visible on seals, No. 4 and 6. All these Paśupati seals do not in any respect closely resemble the priest king statue as stated by Parpola (1981). The sitting posture of Paśupati is totally different from that of the preist king.

Western counterpart of Paśupati.

In the Celtic mythology there is a deity identical with Indian Paśupati. The picture of the diety is engraved on the famous bowl from Gundenstrupp, Jutland. It is the picture of the male god Cernunnos or Lord of the beasts sitting in folded legs position similar to Paśupati but not identical. He is shown to be holding a serpent in the left hand and circular ring in right hand. He is shown to be surrounded by both domestic and fierce animals.

Description of Paśupati seal no. 1

On the seal is depicted the central figure sitting in folded legs position surrounded by animls, starting anticlockwise from the bottom, the first figure is that of a goat (*Apra hircus*) with long curved horns. It is a common species of goat found in the Sind province. It is shown to have turned its head upwards as if it is looking at the central figure. The next figure is that of a common Indian buffalo (*Babalus bubalis*). Above this figure is a figure of the single horned rhinoceros (*Rhinoceros unicornis*) which is obvious because of the single horn projecting from its nose. In the right hand top corner is a human figure but it constitutes a part of graffitti as shown below. In the left top corner is a figure of an Indian elephant (*Elephas maximus linnaeus*) with its trunk directed downwards. Then follows the human figure and the last being the tiger (*Panthera tigris*). The bottom left corner is broken. However, in the bottom centre mirror image of the goat horns is clearly visible.

The central figure is highly decorated with ornaments on chest. The protruding breasts and large belly portion, both the convincing signs of mother godess are absent.

AV II 34 and the Paśupati seal

The deity Pasupati is absent in the ṚV lore. It occurs several times in VS text and the AV text. There is no separate deity Paśupati in VS but it is one of the epithets of the Rudra who is again a Ṛgvedic deity. He is referred to as god of the beasts and Mahādeva as well. In AV also the term Paśupati is an epithet of Rudra. However the hymn II. 34 is devoted to Paśupati as separate entity. The seal describes the total theme of the hymn. The hymn is ascribed to the seer Atharvā. Whitney points out that it was recited during sacrifice of an animal. All the five stanzas of the hymns throw light on the seal. They are given below with explanatory comments. (Whitney 1905).

(Translation by Whitney)

ya iśe paśupatiḥ paśūnām
catuṣpādāmuta yo dvipadam
niṣkrītaḥ sa yajñiyam bhāgametu rāyaspoṣā
yajamānam sacantām | | AV II. 34.

Tr: "The lord of the cattle, who rules over (iṣ) the cattle, the four footed and who also rules over the two footed - let him, bought off, go to (his) sacrificial portion, let abundance of wealth attach themselves to (sac) the sacrificer".

As described in the stanza, the Passupati, lord of the beasts is lord of both the quadruped and the biped living beings, confirming the figures inscribed on the seal.

The theme would have been incomplete without a separate human figure, a biped, as shown below the elephant. Thus the human figure inscribed in the right hand top corner should be part of the graffitti and not the pictorial representation.

pramuñcato bhuvanasya reto gātum
dhatta yagamānāya devāḥ.
upākṛtam śaśamānam yadastātpriyam
devānāmapyetu pāthaḥ. AV II. 34.2.

Tr: "Do ye, releasing (pra-muc) the seed of being, assign progress (gatu) to the sacrificer, O Gods, what hath stood brought hither (upākṛta) strenous (śaśamāna); let it go upon the dear path of the Gods".

The central . deity is in the state of phallus erectum as if he is about to release semen - the seed of the universe. The sitting posture of the Paśupati is also significant. He is sitting in the Yonyāsana posture with slight variation. In this yoga posture, the performer folding his legs at knees arranges soles to face each other making an appear-ance of pudenda. It is evident from the Paśupati figure. Thus both the parts of the human body associated with the act of procreation are shown in the figure confirming the epithet of "bhuvanasya retaḥ", i.e. seed of the universe or creation.

ye badhyamānamanu dīdhyānā
anvaikṣanta manasā cakṣuṣā ca.
agnistānagre pra mumoktu devo
viśvakarmā prajayā samrarāṇaḥ | | AV II. 34.3

Tr: "They, who giving attention to (anudhi) the one being bound, looked after (him) with mind and eye-let the divine Agni at first (agre) release them, he the all working, in unison with (saṁ-rā) progeny".

All the animals except the elephant in the left top corner are shown to be gazing at the central figure. He too can be imagined to be looking at them with the mind and eyes. It is possible only while meditating in yogic trance. The Paśupati is looking at his own creation with compassionate look through omnispread vision and omnipresent mind in yogic trance. The animals too are in unison with him. However, variation in the pose of an elephant cannot be explaied.

ye grāmyaḥ paśavo viśvarūpā virūpāḥ
santo bahudhaikarūpāḥ.
vāyuṣṭānagre pramumoktu devaḥ prajāpatiḥ
prajayā samrarāṇaḥ. AV II. 34.4

Tr: "cattle that are of the village, all formed being of various forms, manifolding of one form - let the divine Vāyu at first release them, Prajāpati in unison with progeny.

This stanza points to the distinction between the domestic bovine -animals i.e. grāmyaḥ and the wild or forest animals. While commenting on this stanza Whitney points out that the black Yajus Text TS III. 1 is the same hymn except the change in the order of stanzas. It has only slight variation in the text, i.e. āraṇyāḥ - of the forest - being substituted for grāmyāḥ. This substitution perfectly matches with the animals engraved on the seal. Both the types of animals being progeny his other epithet being Prajāpati.

Prajānantaḥ pratim gṛṇhantu pūrve
prāṇamaṅgebhyaḥ paryācarantam.
divam gaccha prati tiṣṭhā śarīraiḥ
svargam yāhi pathibhirdevayānaiḥ. AV II. 34.5

Tr: "For knowing, let them first (pūrva) receive the breath (prāṇa) coming to them forth from limbs. Go to heaven, stand firm with thy bodies, go to paradise (svarga) by God travelled roads."

The last stanza ordains the sacrifical animals to travel along the path of gods. This also explains why the animals are gazing towards Paśupati.

Reference to rectangular seal

The deity on the seal being Paśupati, it was an epithet of Rudra as in VS and AV texts. VS describes Rudra as the one with blue neck (VS XVI. 8 and others). Similarly epithet Mahādeva is also used in connection with the Paśupati (VS XXIX. 8) Thus Rudra - Śiva - Mahādeva - Paśupati represent the same deity in the AV and VS lore, that continued in the later times, while the AV hymn refers to only quadruped and biped animals, the reptiles like snake are absent. May be because it was not a sacrifical animal. However, all these animals are mentioned in AV XI. 2.24-25 where the plaits of Paśupati -Rudra are also referred in AV XI 2.31.

In the later day mythology, the deity Śiva-Mahādeva always had cobra around his neck. This association dates back to the Indus culture times as indicated by the rectangular seal legend in seal No. 4. Here the central deity is seated in Pasupati's pose and flanked on both the sides by a devotee sitting on either side and also a cobra in hood spread position. Thus the deity on the Paśupati seal is Rudra - Mahādeva deity in formative stage. As such, the VS points to his blue neck, around which the myth of drinking poison was woven. Or was it already in circulation during the Indus period as a part of tradition?

Positive animals in the left hand corner of seal no.1

This most important seal i.e. No. 1 is unfortunately broken However, it is now possible to contemplate the possible animal types engraved in the broken corner. The biped animal belonging to the bird species and a quadruped animal like lizard or amphiba animal like crocodile might have been engraved on the broken portion of the seal. This is further confirmed by the seal No. 7 where the central deity is flanked by fish, crocodile and snakes.

Conclusions

The methodology of drawing parallels can be successfully applied to the Vedic and post Vedic culture in India to understand the Indus culture.

The mother goddess cult as practised in the West probably did not exist in the Indus culture.

The terracotta female figures from the Indus culture need not be the virgin goddesses but terracotta toys for the female kids.

Horned headgear was the prerogative of male deity or male human figures engraved on the Indus seals. However, long plaits or bun did not definitely point to the female sex. Both the male and female could be having plaits.

The cylindrical seal from Kalibangan does not depict the scene of virgin sacrifice and the fire altars at Kalibangan may not be the vestal fires as proposed by Atre.

The famous Paśupati seal can be better understood in the light of the Atharva Vedic hymn II. 34. He is the Lord of beasts and presides over all types of animals, namely domestic and fierce, wild, cervix, amphibians and aqatic animals.

It is hoped that the Ṛgvedic and the Atharva Vedic lore shall be explored further as this can help to understand the Indus culture and religion.

REFERENCES

Agrawal, P.K. 1984. *Goddesses in Ancient India.* Abhinav Publications, Delhi. Plates Illustrating various mother Goddess statues.

Atre, Shubhangana. 1986. Lady of Beasts: The Harappan Goddess. *Purtattava.* 16: 7-14.

Casal, J.M. 1961. *Fouilles De Mundigak* Paris I and II. Plate XXXII A-B and Fig. 64.

Fentress, Marcia. 1979. Indus charms and Urns: A look at religious diversity at Harappa and Mohenjodaro. *Man and Environment.* VII: 102.

Jarrige, J.F. and M. Lechevallier, 1977. *Excavations at Mehergarh* Baluchistan: Their significance in the perhistorical context of Indo-Pakistan Boarderlands. *South Asian Archaeology.* 1977: 463-535.

Leroi-Gourhan A. 1968. *The Art of Prihistoric man in Western Europe.* London: 113.

Macay, E.J.H., 1938 *Further Excavations at Mohenjodaro.* 2 Vols. Govt. of India. New Delhi.

Marshall, John. 1931. *Mohenjodaro and the Indus Civilizaiton.* 3 Vols. London: A Probsthain.

Marshall, J. 1931. *Mohenjodaro and Indus civilization.* III. PL CXI: 357

New Larousse Encyclopedia of Mythology 1987 Hamlyn England: 224.

Pandeya, Rajabali. 1978. *Hindu Dharm Kosh (Hindi).* U.P. Hindi Samsthan Lucknow: 696.

Parpola, Asko. 1985. The Sky Garment, *Studies Oriental.* 57 :12-013.

Parpola, Asko. 1981. New Correspondences between Harappan and Near Eastern Glyptic Art, A paper read at the 6th Conf. of South Asian Archaeology held at Cambridge 5-10 July 1981 and also reprinted with some modifications in South Asian Archaeology (1981): 176-05.

Piggot, Stuart. 1961. *Prehistoric India.* Pelican books Fig. 9 on 108.

Sullivan, H.P. A Re-examination of the religion of the Indus civilization, *History of religion. Ed.* Mercea Eliada et al. Chicago (1): 115-125.

Thapar, B.K. 1973. Synthesis of the multiple data as obtained from Kalibangan. *Radio carbon dating and Indian Archaeology.* Ed. D.P. Agrawal and A. Ghosh. T.I.F.R. Bombay :264-271.

Thapar, B.K. 1979. *Kalibangan: A Harappan Metropolis* beyond *the Indus Valley,* Ancient cities of the Indus, Ed. G.L. Possehl: 196-202. PL XXIII.

Vats, M.S. 1940. *Excavations at Harappa.* 2 Vols. Govt. of India. Delhi.

Wheeler, REM. 1966. *Civilizaitons of the Indus* Valley *and Beyond* Thames and Hudson. London: 34-35.

Vats, M.S. 1940. *Excavations at Harappa.* PL 39:305.

Whitney, W.D. 1905. *Atharva Veda Samhita (Translation).* Harvard Oriental series.

Defence System in Ancient India, based on Literary and Archaeological Evidence

V.C. SHARMA*

The idea of defence led the man to experiment with various means of protection and in the long run he organized an elaborate machinery of defence system (Dikshitar 1948:25). Insecurity invites security which compelled man to live in groups close to each other. These small settlements lying in areas of attraction later developed in the shape of towns by way of trade or political authority. In the beginning, the security of these places started with a simple fortification but later on other defensive features were added in the form of moat, bastions, high towers etc. with further compartmentalization by way of adding inner fortification walls. The military aspects of the forts cannot be denied completely. It may be added here that in the present paper the discussion is confined only upto Gupta period and only those examples have been quoted which have bearing on the development phases of defence system in ancient India.

Literary Sources

The Vedic and Brahmana literature including Arthashastra and Niti-Shastra provide ample references. The art of fortification had already advanced much prior to Vedic Aryans, and in Rigveda, there is description of forts belonging to pre-Aryan inhabitants, called *Dasas* or *Dasyus*. The words for rampart, fort and stronghold or defence wall have been termed in Rigveda as *Pura* (R.V. I. 53, 7; 58, 8; 131, 4; iii 15, 4; iv 27, 1), *Durga (R.V. V. 7; vii.* 25, 2) *and Dehi* (R.V. vi. 47, 2 vii 6,5). A fort with a hundred walls called *Satabhuji* is mentioned in Rigveda (R.V. 1. 66, 8; vii 15, 14). The later Brahmanas and Upanishads, refer *Pura (Aitareya Brahmana* I. 23, II 11; *Chhandogya Upanishad* viii. 5:3) and *Mahapur (Gopatha Brahmana.* ii. 2:7), meaning rampart or fort and a great fortress respectively. Manu *(Manu Samhita.* Chap. VII, 70-75) speaks of the variety of forts i.e. with deserts on all the sides, with water all around, with rampart around, surrounded by thorny plants, made of elephants, horses, infantry etc. and fort on a hill. In his *Astadhyai,* Panini refers to rampart *(prakara),* moat *(parikha)* and gates *(dwara)* as important parts of the city for the purpose of its defence.

Jatakas refer the cities being fortified with walls and ramparts, with buttresses, watch towers and massive gates (Chakravarti 1941: 128). The city of Vaisali had a triple wall around it alongwith gates and watch-tower (Cowell 1957 Jataka. I. 316). Similarly the cities of Mithila (Cowell 1957: Jataka, VI, 30) and Potali (Cowell 1957: Jataka. III. 2) had their walls, gates and battlements.,

The art of fortification had highly developed by the time of Kautilya, who considered the fort as one of the seven constituent elements of the State (Chakravarti 1941: 134). He has enumerated four kinds of forts (Arthashastra. B.K. II. Chap. III) viz. hill fort *(parvata),* water fort *andaka,* desert fort *(dhanvana)* and forest fort *(vanadurga).* He further prescribes rules regarding construction of forts i.e., its shape, circular or rectangular or square being dictated by the nature of ground and whether it should be surrounded by three successive ditches or moats. He has given various details regarding the set-up of inner part of the fort. He also gives a list of various immovable machines - *Sthirayantras (Arthashastra.* B.K. II. Chap. 18) which seem to have been specially stored in forts to

* Archaeological Survey of India, Janpath, New Delhi.

repulse attacks. Most of the weapons of the offence were also used for defence. There were weapons exclusively for defence and these arms include mainly shield and body armour (Chakravati 1941: 175).

Some kind of body armour was known to the Vedic people. The term Kavacha in the sense of a breast-plate occurs in *Atharvaveda* (Atharvaveda XI. 10.22). The metal armour is also mentioned by Brahmanas. *(Jaiminiya Upanishad Brahmana* IV: 1. 3) Describing the battle of Hydaspes Arrian (Mc Crindle 1974: 108) refers to the armour, which Porus was wearing and says that it was 'shot proof'. Rigveda mentions arm-guard as *Hastaghna* (R.V. VI. 75, 14) which was used by the archer to protect his hand from the blow of string while shooting arrow.

Kautilya *(Arthashastra* B.K. II. Chap. 18) has used the term Avarna for the shield and Varma for body armours. About the shields he says, *Peti* (basketry), *carma* (leather shield), *Hastikarna* (elephants ear), *Talamula,* Dhamanika (bladder), *Kavata* (doorwing) and *Kitika* (light shield) are the instruments used in self defence. These defensive arms were made of leather wood, creepers and bamboo etc. The body armour was also used apart from the shield for the purpose of defence while fighting. Several varieties of armour were made of horns and skins as is evident from *Arthashastra.* The animals, whose horns and skins were used for armour were tortoise, rhinoceros, bison, elephant and cow. The body armours were also fabricated out of the iron net *(loha-jala),* little iron-net *(loha-jalika)* iron plate garments *(loha-patta* and iron armour *(kavacha).*

The armours were not only used by men but the war elephants and war horses were also protected from the attack of the enemies army.

Fortifications and moats around cities are described in literature (Ghosh 1973: 62). No defence exists at Charsada, ancient *Puskalavati,* but their prior existence is assumed, as the surviving account of Alexander's maneuver hereabouts in 327 B.C. shows, that a trusted general with a division of his troops took 30 days to reduce the town, which justifies that the place was fortified (Wheeler 1962:5).

Archaeological Data

The system of defence as described in the ancient literature was also confirmed by the archaeological evidences. However, the archaeological evidences put the defence system to more hoary past than what we get in literature.

Pre-Harappan and Harappan Defences

At Kalibangan both the pre-Harappan and Harappan settlements were fortified (Thapar 1975:20-23; 1976: 5-8). The excavations at Kalibangan brought into light a pre-Harappan fortification wall made of mud bricks, upon which Harappan fortification itself rests at certain points. This shows that the time when the Harappan fortification wall was erected, the Pre-Harappan one had already gone into disuse and at places a new wall was constructed upon the old one after giving fresh facing. The single gateway in the pre-Harappan fortification in the northern wall towards the north-west is just a passage which had direct and easy entry from the outside. No guard room, control tower or stair case has been found attached to any of the gateway.

The citadel complex at Kalibangan was not just one unit, with a single outline, but consisted of two parts, a southern and a northern. Each part was in the form of a rhomb, and enclosed by a fortification wall and bastions. There was a common wall (bipartite wall) in between. In the case of bipartite wall, however, two central salients projected into the area of the northern rhomb which clearly indicates that the construction belong to southern rhomb and not to the northern (Lal 1984: 56). The citadel at kalibangan is more or less akin to that of Harappa.

The excavations at Kot Diji (Pakistan Archaeology No. 1, 1964: 40-41) in West Pakistan brought into light a fortification wall in the levels preceding Harappan occupation. This fortification wall is built on bed-rock with undressed courses of lime-stone blocks having a mud-brick super structure and strengthened externally with bastions at irregular intervals, further supported by a mud brick revetment on the outside. In Upper Kot Diji phase, the fortifications fell in disuse even in the life time of Kot Dijian who used its top for occupational purposes (Dikshit 1980: 42).

Apart from Kot Diji and Kalibangan, there are a few other sites viz. Khotras Buthi, Tharro and Dhillanijo Kot all in sind (Piggott 1950: 77, 78) where remains of early fortifications were found.

The mode of defence continued in the form of fortification in the phase succeeding the Pre-Harappan and most interesting evidence comes from the famous site of Harappa. The excavations here by Wheeler (Ancient India No. 30 1947: 64-66) revealed that the defence on plan enclosed an area in the shape of a parallelogram with rectangular salients or towres, some of which rising higher than the wall, at fairly frequent intervals. The excavations further revealed that a mud-brick wall with a basal width of about 14m and rising with a taper to a height of over 12 m. went round the mound (Lal 1984: 55). The cutting across the defence revealed a rampart of mud and mud-bricks and on this rampart stood the main mud-brick defensive wall with battered exterior. The defences show three periods of construction. After a long period of weathering and other damage, the original baked revetment was rebuilt, particularly in the north-west corner where it was considerably thickened. In the third phase, the north-west corner tower was reinforced by a new tower.

At Mohenjodaro the possibility of tower walls was pointed out by Marshall and Mackey in earlier excavations. Wheeler (1953: 27) after a limited field work has shown the possibility of defences on the citadel mound. Near the south-east corner a system of solid burnt-brick towers was exposed. The tower stood on the massive burnt-brick towers was exposed. The tower stood on the massive burnt-brick foundations and was originally reinforced by horizontal timbers. Two of the towers on the south-east corner seemed to have been flanked by a postern gate which was blocked at some later stage. On the western side of the citadel, a high baked brick tower was partially uncovered. To the north of this tower a small postern has been identified.

Banawali is another fortified town of the Harappans. The defensive wall ranges in width from 5.40 to 7.50 m. and segregates the citadel from the rest of the town which in turn spreads out in the east as well as north. It is a fortified town with an additional citadel inside. thus dividing the whole township, into two parts i.e. the Citadel (Acropolis) and lower town. Both the divisions have enormous defensive walls and have been provided with entry-points and extensive bastions. The citadel at Banawali (Bisht 11984: 91-93) is located inside the township, making it a key point of the whole scheme. So is the case at Balu excavated by Kurukshetra University (*IAR* 1982-83).

Another Harappan settlement is Surkotada where surrounding walls with gateways have been found (Joshi 1966: 64; Joshi 1972: 98-144). Kesarvani has made a special study of Harappan gateways (kesarvani 1984: 63). The characteristic feature of the fortification is that alongwith mud and mud-bricks, rubble was also used for its construction *(IAR* 1970-71: 71: 13; *IAR* 1971-72).

In the earliest phase IA at Surkotada, two gateways of mud and mud-bricks were noticed, out of which one is located on the south-western side of eastern fortification wall while the other on the souther side of the citadel area, fronting the gateway complex of phase IC (Joshi 1972: 122). The gateways were rebuilt in stone during phase IC. A gateway complex with 10x23 m projection was built on the southern fortification wall of the citadel *(IAR* 1971-72: 18). Two guard rooms one either side were erected on the fortification wall.

Lothal *(IAR* 1955-56: 13) has revealed three main periods of occupation called pre-defence, defence and post defence periods. The earliest occupation before the erection of defences suffered damage from the floods of the Bhogavo and Sabarmati rivers. This necessitated the erection of a huge solid mud platform of mud bricks. Considering the height as safe from floods, people built their dwellings on the platform. With the experience of subsequent floods they raised the height of mud platform and erected a clay rampart in addition, ushering in the defence period. The rampart appeared to have been quite wide and high. It was meant as a defence against floods, is proved by the traces of frequent breaches, the repairs and reinforcements provided to it and flood deposits of debris and silt. As a last alternate the northern phase of the platform was reverted with bricks and a major breach was emend by the erection of a buttress-wall behind the breach and filling up the intermediate space with mud.

The evidence of fortification of this period may also be gathered from various other sites viz. Ali Murad in Sind, Sutakagen-Dor and Sutka Koh in Makran.

At Desalpur *(IAR* 1963-64: 10-12) a massive stone fortification with a basal width of 4 m, rising to an extant height of 2.5 m was found. The fortification wall was reinforced with corner towers and salients. The north-eastern corner showed an additional feature of mud brick filling in the shape of a platform, between the outer and inner stone veneer-wallings. For the habitation inside the town, many houses were built against the fort wall itself (Soundara Rajan: 1977).

Chalcolithic Defences

The rampart at Eran *(IAR* 1962-63: 11), 6.40 m in extent height was found to have been 47 m in basal width. Built of black and yellow clay, the core material contained pottery of the same series as that of the Chalcolithic occupation. The fortified settlement was girdled on three sides by the Bina river and on the fourth being south, a moat 36.57 m in width and 5.28 m in depth. The antiquity of the fortification is a debatable issue and it may not be earlier than the beginning of the Historic period.

Nagda *(IAR* 1955-56: 14) has revealed massive mudbricks structures, the possibility of one of these being a ramp bastion cannot be ruled out.

Defence Plans of the Historical Period

The beginning of historical period witnessed rise of sixteen *Mahajanapadas,* all having well fortified capital cities. Excavations at some of these sites viz. Ahichchhatra, Kausambi, Rajghat, Rajgir, Sravasti, Vaisali, Ujjain etc. have revealed fortification, which, in initial stages are same at all the sites i.e. a mud rampart with moat around it. In the later stages brick walls were added to the rampart. There were other fortified cities in East Indian such as Chandraketugarh in 24-Parganas.

At Ahichchhatra there were two phases of rampart enclosing the city wall with a perimeter of about 6 kms and had a brick wall with 'boxes' at the top. In the subsequent excavations in (1963-65), the mud rampart was seen to belong to Kaushana times (*IAR* 1963-64: 44).

A massive burnt brick Kushana wall perhaps for the defence was found at Hulas. The main wall was having a width of about 2.10 m end the size of the bricks used therein was 52x28x8 cm. The height of the wall was approximately 1.80 m, with 18 brick courses. The east-west arm of the wall was about 52 m long while the north-south 30 m. The wall at the corner was roundish, and a rectangular platform was projecting from the inner side of the roundish corner which was perhaps a part of a bastion. The remains of an entrance gate and a few drains as a part of this wall were also found (Dikshit 1981: 71-72).

The extensive boundary wall at Kausambi (*IAR* 1955-56: 20) with brick revetment erected to enclose the entire monastery. The wall was of lesser width in norther, eastern and western sides in comparison to southern side, which was much wider. A wide pavement flanked the southern wing. Two parallel walls were also erected in the south-eastern and south-western corners of monastery for enclosing two newly built stupas by rectangular enclosures.

A mud rampart about 5 km in circuit, later on topped by a burnt brick wall was found at Sravasti, which was built in early phase of period II (c. 275 to 200 B.C.).

At Ujjain (*IAR* 1955-56: 19) to save the city from destruction the first settlers on the site erected a massive mud wall of compact whitish clay laid in bands, separated by sticky dark clay with charcoal. Owing to the relentless floods, the rampart even to its upper parts suffered badly and only patches of it were found in excavations. Timber enforcements are also evident from Ujjain.

At Tilaurakot in Nepalese Tarai a mud rampart was erected in Period II which began in Circa 200 B.C. and it was provided with a brick wall on its outer slopes. (Ghosh 1973: 65).

The great wall of the ancient city of Rajgir completely enclosed the town twenty five to thirty miles running along the hill crest. The wall had square bastions attached to the exterior. During the course of excavations, a mud rampart associated with a moat of uncertain dimensions was revealed. The town is enclosed by an inner fortification wall, which most probably served the purpose of inner line of defence.

The city of imperial Mauryas, Patliputra had an ideal location, surrounded by the rivers Ganga in the north, Punpun on the east and the Son on the south and west. Alongwith this natural line of defence the second line of defence comprised of mud ramparts and towers. Another line of defence existed at a distance of a Kilometre with the ramparts, consisting of ditches, beyond which stood might wooden palisades guarding a brick wall.

Sisupalgarh is a well planned fortified settlement with a peculiar gate complex. The fort on plan is roughly square, with two gateways on each side and four corner towers while the river surrounding the fort with a constant water supply to it. The fortification consists of a rampart, crowned by a double brick wall, the space being filled-up by mud. The gate is of double system the outer and the inner respectively. The outer gate is provided with guard rooms and auxiliary passage. A similar fort could also be seen at Jaugada.

The fortification wall at Nagarjunakonda encloses a trapezoidal shaped area. The burnt-brick wall is built here over the mud rampart. Leaving the portion of the hill, the wall is surrounded by a dith. Out of that three gateways on the east, north and west, the northern one was most probably an emergency exit.

The fortification at Sirkap now in Pakistan is having square bastions projecting frequently at irregular intervals. The main gate is in the northern side and it does not face directly the main street, but turn slightly to the east. The gateway house is comprised of a large hall with guard rooms. The plan of Sirsukh consists of an irregular rectangle. The fortification wall is having a heavy plinth provided on the exterior face, at its base. Semi-circular bastions are erected at regular intervals. The walls and bastions both have loopholes for the use of inmates.

The description of the forts remains incomplete without taking into account the figure of a fort carved in the sculptural panel at Sanchi. Here the depiction of the ancient city of Kusinagara has been made. It shows a wall having battlements with pierced holes for archers. At the corner is an octagonal tower. The wall is double projected on either side of the gateway and the whole fortification is surrounded by a moat. A bridge over the moat is the access to the gate.

Defence Weapons

Before discussing the other aspect of defence, it may be pointed out, that all the weapons used in aggression, were also the arms for defence according to the requirement of circumstances.

The arms which were used only for defence, were very few in number, out of which particular mention may be made of shields which have been represented in the sculptures at various places. For instance in the back of the lower architrave of the southern gateway at Sanchi, scene of the war of relic has been depicted. In this scene the soldiers have been shown holding long shields. Similarly in the friezes of Ranigumpha, Udayagiri hills, Orissa (Majumdar 1936: 78), the representation of warrior with shield may be noticed. Two types of shields may be recognized here according to their size i.e. one smaller than the other. The later are worn by fort soldiers and former by horse-men (Dikshitar 1948: 135). Apart from sculptures, the representation of shield and warriors can be seen in the paintings. Besides other weapons of aggression, the warrior with shields are depicted in the rock paintings of Mahadeo hills (Gordon 1936: 35-41). In Ajanta murals, three types of shields may be noticed. Apart from the crescent and oblong type of shield, a typical shield appeared which resembles with the segment of a wheel, with the spokes left out. It may be the round kind of shield with grotesque forms of tufts or tassels round the fringes thrown over behind the shoulder with strap and buckles (Dikshitar 1948: 138).

Some of the Indo-Scythian coins represent the king wearing coat of mail or chain-armour and helmets. One of the coins of Antimachus represents him holding a trident in his right hand and perhaps a shield hanging from his left.

Conclusion

In nutshell, the above is a brief survey of defence system evolved in Ancient India. In the beginning it was a simple fortification which later on became complex due to necessities. The early fortifications were meant against the neighbourers or other barbaric societies, but in due course these very groups became organized and it was not possible for these simple fortified villages to sustain the organized hoards merely by a defence wall. As the concept of state came in vogue, more radical steps were taken to safeguard the capital-cities from the invasions, this is how the defence system developed in medieval times.

REFERENCES

Ancient India 3. 1947. Delhi.

Bisht, R.S. 1984. Structural Remains and Town-Planning of Banawali. *Frontriers of the Indus Civilization.* New Delhi.

Chakravarti, P.C. 1941. *The Art of War in Ancient India.*

Cowell, E.B. 1957. *Jataka. Cambridge.*

Dikshitar, R.V.V. 1948. *War in Ancient India.*

Dikshit, K.N. 1980. A Critical Review of the Pre-Harappan Cultures. *Man and Environment.* IV. Ahmedabad.

Dikshit, K.N. 1981. The excavations at Hulas and further exploration of the Upper Ganga-Yamuna doab. *Man and Environment.* V. Pune.

Ghosh, A. 1973. *The City in Early Historical India.* Simla.

Gordon, D.H. 1936. The Rock Paintings of the Mahadeo Hills. *Indian Arts and Letters.* X. 1. London.

Indian Archaeology 1955-56 *A Review,* 1962-63 *A Review* 1963-64 *A Review,* 1970-71 *A Review,* 1971-72 *A Review,* 1982-83 *A Review.*

Joshi, J.P. 1966. Exploration in Norther Kutch. *Journal of Oriental Institute.* Baroda; 16. 1: 62-69.

Joshi, J.P. 1972. Exploration in Kutch and Excavations at Surkotada and New Light on the Harappan Migration. *Journal of Oriental Institute. Baroda.* 22. 1-2: 98-144.

Kesarvani, A. 1984 Harappan Gateways: A functional reassessment. *Frontriers of the Indus Civilization.* New Delhi.

Lal, B.B. 1984. Some Reflections on the structural remains at Kalibanga. *Frontriers of the Indus Civilization.* New Delhi.

Macdonell, A.A. and A.B. Keith. 1912. *Vedic Index of Names and Subjects* London.

Majumdar, N.G. 1936. *A Guide to the Sculptures in Indian Museum.* I. Delhi.

Mc. Crindle, J.W. 1974. *The invasion of India by Alexander The Great. Pakistan Archaeology.* 1. 1964. Karachi.

Piggott, S. 1950. *Pre-Historic India.* Harmondsworth.

Soundara Rajan, K.V. 1977. Kutch Harappan. *The Indus Civilization: Problem and Issue.* Simla. (Cyclostyled paper).

Thapar, B.K. 1975. Kalibangan: A Harappan Metropolis Beyond the Indus Valley. *Expedition.* 17. 2:19-32.

Thaper, B.K. 1976. The Concept of the Citadel in the Indus Civilization. *30th International Congress of Human Sciences in Asia and North Africa.* Mexico (Cyclostyled paper).

Wheeler, R.E.M. 1953. *The Indus Civilization.* London

Wheeler, R.E.M. 1962. *Charsada.* Oxford.

NOTES AND NEWS

On the Decipherment of the Indus Script by Soviet Scholars*

A team of Soviet scholars led by Yu. V. Knorozov has been systematically engaged in the decipherment of the Indus script for over two decades. They have so far brought out six collections of their studies in this series the first of which was published in 1965. While Yu. V. Knorozov has mainly done the formal analysis of the Indus texts, the linguistic analysis has been done by N.V. Gurov and M.F. Albedil. B. Ya. Volchok has dealt with the astronomical aspect on the basis of the Indus texts. The positional-statistical analysis was done by A.M. Kondratov. Some other Soviet scholars have also participated in this project: G.V. Aleksyeyev, M.A. Probst, I.K. Fyodorova and V.M. Misyugin. It is worth mentioning that the Soviets have given some detailed readings of the Indus signs and texts only in their latest publication *PROTO-INDICA:* 1979, Moscow, 1981.

The Indus script has been considered as morphemic-syllabic type of hieroglyphic writing. The language of the Indus people belonged to the Dravidian family of languages. The Soviets call this language as 'Proto-Indian'.

The Soviet scholars have come to a firm conclusion with regard to the structure of the Indus text-signs, i.e. signs as used in the texts. Most of the signs occur in such a way that they form blocks. A block is a group of signs which is repeated in many inscriptions.

Within a block there is a constant sign which stands for the root. Other signs in a block are variable and semi-variable signs. They can occur before or after the constant sign. In a block there can be more than one root-sign. A constant sign can also be used as initial semi-variable in some other block. Root-signs with short vertical strokes on both sides have been called as circumgraphs. A number of signs have two or more variants. These characteristics of the Indus text-signs have been explained in all the publications of the Soviet team.

Linguistic affinity of the Proto-Indian language has been determined on the basis of the formal analysis of the Indus text-signs. The language of the Indus texts has agglutinative features and has no prefixes which conforms to the structure of the Dravidian languages. The blocks in the Indus texts represent word-forms in which the first sign stands for the root followed by postfixes. These postfixes are of two types: the derivative (word-building) suffixes and the grammatical (form-building) markers.

The agglutinative character of the language of the Indus script has been illustrated by the following example:

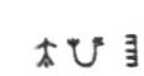

āṇ-or-at[tu]-kā

'to the respected God-warrior'

Here *āṇ*  'warrior' is the root, *or* is the plural suffix used in the sense of Pluralis honorificus, *at[tu]*  is the suffix of the oblique case, and *kā*  is the suffix of the dative case.

Although the Indus script is written from right to left all the readings have been given from left to right as in *Proto-Indica* 1979. The signs incorporated in this paper have been copied from the Russian text.

* Paper read at the seminar organized by the Bihar Puravid Parishad, Patna, 18-19, October, 1986.

In the agglutinative languages the position of affixes - prefixes, postfixes etc. - is strictly fixed which has been mentioned by the Soviet scholars also. Moreover, the agglutinative languages use standard affixes and the same markers - plural markers, masculine markers, feminine markers etc. - are used in all the parts of speeches wherever there is such distinction *(Introduction to Linguistics* (in Russian) Reformatsky, A.A., Moscow., 1961: 270-272). The decipherment as proposed by the Soviet team in many cases does not satisfy both these conditions.

The sign / denoting form-building postifix can combine with the sign U and can change places with it in ligature U| This is a contradiction of what has been said about the fixed place of postfixes in agglutinative languages." After the root or the word-building semi-variable (when there is one) come the variable signs of 1st positional group |, U, ヨ denoting form-building postfixes; sign / . (identical to figure 1 and the non-notional initial variable) can combine with the sign U, 'U' and, moreover it can change places with it (in ligature U|)" *PROTO-INDICA:* 1979, p. 10). Postfixes can form chains with hierarchic sequence from one to several parts, with their position vis-a-vis one another strictly fixed." *(PROTO-INDICA. 1979*: p. 17).

More examples can be given from the proposed deciherment where strict order of writing has not been followed although the sign conveys one and the same meaning. The same figure / which has been deciphered as *or* denoting Pluralis honorificus as a homonym occurs in three different positions in the same meaning:

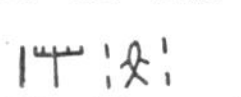
or per nal min
'our great good star'

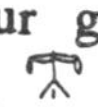
kā-or
'honoured protector'

mā-or
'honoured black [god]

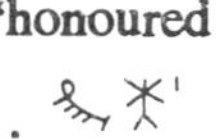
sir amma-or
'honoured lady of buffalo'

(PROTO-INDICA. 1979: 64, 65).

The number |||| has been deciphered as *nal* meaning 'good' as a homonym. In this meaning the sign |||| occurs also as a circumgraph:

nal min
'good star'

nal mur
'good youth'

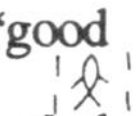
nal ke
'good red [god]

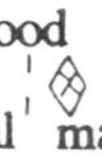
nal mari
'good rain'

(*PROTO-INDICA*: 1979: p. 68)

If these signs have one and the same meaning there is no apparent difficulty in writing them in one and the same position.

We also find that the Proto-Indian postfixes as deciphered by Soviet scholars are not standard postfixes which is necessary for a language to be called agglutinative. For example, three different plural markers have been identified: | , ヨ , and U
All of them have been given three different readings:

/ or
ヨ ka
U aḷ

In an agglutinative language the plural postfix as a grammatical marker should have the same phonetic reading with some positional variations. If all these signs are plural markers then their different readings (and also different ways of writing) goes against the features of agglutinative languages.

Our observations on the decipherment of the Indus script by Soviet scholars are in no way an assessment of their important work. Segmentation of the Indus text-signs into blocks is a significant step forward in the formal analysis of the Indus script. The proposed decipherment and other interpretations have to be reviewed by experts from different fields.

Centre of Russian Studies
Jawaharlal Nehru University, New Delhi.

HEM CHANDRA PANDE

Anangpur: A Paleolithic Site near Delhi

The Paleolithic site of Anangpur (28° 27′30" N, 77° 15′56" E), Distt. Faridabad (Haryana), is located 30 kms. south of Delhi beyond Surajkund on the quartzite tableland of Tuglakabad-Gurgaon area which attains a height of about 243 m. above sea level and nearly 30 m. above the surface of the present plain. It lies in between the fourth and fifth palaeochannels of Yamuna. Indications are that the river's fifth shift eastwards was around late Pleistocene era. It is therefore natural that the tools found are mostly of late Acheulian period.

The site which was discovered in 1986 revealed

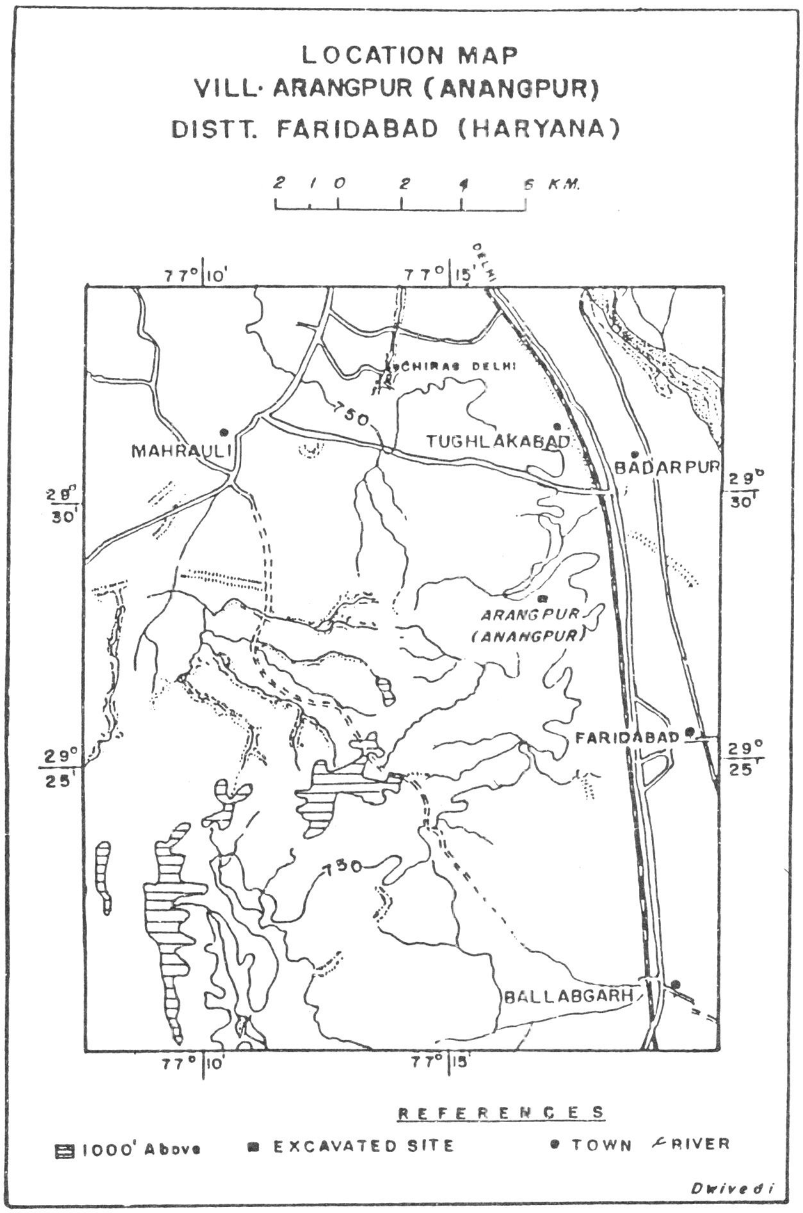

large number of late Acheulian tools from the surface as well from the sections exposed due to quarrying for Badarpur sand.

In the summer of 1991, the area around Anangpur was put to extensive investigation. In order to ascertain the position of the implementiferous horizon in the area, a small trench 3 x 3 m. was taken up. The trench was excavated upto the level of top of bed-rock. As available in the exposed sections, tool bearing layer was encountered just above the bedrock, at a depth of 0.75 m. from the surface. This depth varies from place to place depending on the undulating surface of the bedrock and the deposit over it. The thickness of the implementiferous deposit also varies, ranging from 0.25 to 0.40 m. Just over the implementiferous layer 0.10 m. thick layer of whitish compact clay runs throughout and is the actual sealing layer. The thick deposit of sand and soil over it is the material obtained from the decomposed rocks and erosional activity.

The stone tools (pl. XXV) recovered from Anangpur area are mostly made of fine grained quartzite except few which are on sandstone. The raw material exploited are from the exposed outcrops in the area. The artefacts of quartzite are slightly weathered (patinated) whereas sandstone ones exhibit moderate weathering. The stone tool assemblage comprises of mostly, handaxes and cleavers, few choppers, scrapers, picks, points and horse-hoof cores. Apart from these a large number of cores, flakes and waste flakes are also found. Preliminary analysis of handaxes and cleavers (which constitute majority of the finished tools) reveals the assemblage to be of Late Acheulian phase.

The interesting feature noticed among the handaxes is that in most of the cases the working point is broken due to use. Absence of abraded (due to transportation) tools and occurrence of a large amount of waste products such as cores and flakes clearly suggest that the site at Anangpur is a habitational-cum-factory site of Early Man.

Archaeological Survey of India,
Prehistory Branch, Nagpur.

A.K. SHARMA AND S. B. OTA

REFERENCES

Chakrabarti, D.K. and N. Lahiri. 1987. A preliminary report on the stone age of the Union territory of Delhi and Haryana. *Man and Environment.* XI: 109-116.

Grover, A.K. and P.L. Bakliwal. 1985. River migration and the floods - a study of a section of Yamuna river through remote sensing. *Man and Environment.* IX: 151-153.

Pande, B.M. 1985. A late Acheulian handaxe from New Delhi. *Man and Environment.* IX: 157-158.

Sankalia, H.D. 1974. *The Prehistory and Protohistory of India and Pakistan.* Deccan College. Pune.

Excavations at Golabai Sasan, District Puri, Orissa

Village Golabai Sasan Lat. 20° 01′ N Long. 83°.33.05"E, in Puri district is located in the laterite zone and is situated on the left bank of River Mandakini a tributary of the River Daya. The mound is of considerable size and is cut into two halves by a cart track.

Excavations were undertaken by the Excavation Branch-IV of the Archaeological Survey of India.

A trench 5x5 m. was taken on the southern slope of the mound and dug upto a depth of 5.65 m. The top of the trench, being on the slope, was about 2 m. below the top surface of the mound. In all 20 habitational layers were met with and during excavations floor level of red morrum, in the upper layers and of compact clay in lower layers were found in association with post holes. Fairly good quantity of ash deposits bearing pot sherds and tools were found over the floor levels. In the upper levels, the thickness of floor levels was less as compared with those in lower levels. The floors in the lower levels were of yellowish as well as of blueish clay and the quantity of ash over them was also less. The

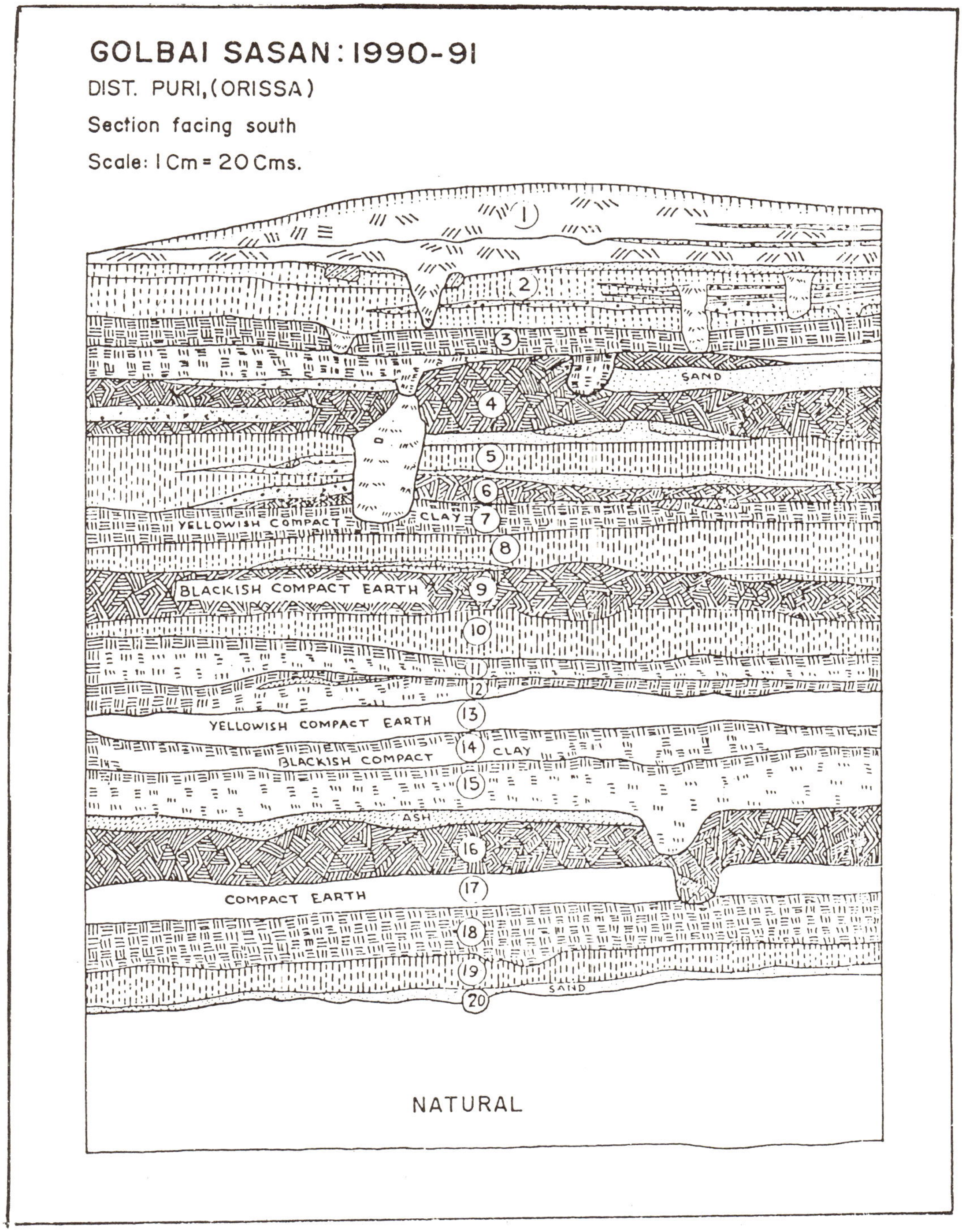
GOLBAI SASAN: 1990-91
DIST. PURI, (ORISSA)
Section facing south
Scale: 1 Cm = 20 Cms.
1
2
3
SAND
4
5
6
YELLOWISH COMPACT CLAY
7
8
BLACKISH COMPACT EARTH
9
10
11
12
YELLOWISH COMPACT EARTH
13
14
BLACKISH COMPACT CLAY
15
ASH
16
COMPACT EARTH
17
18
19
SAND
20
NATURAL

entire deposit, measuring about 5 mt. can be divided into four phases, the pottery of each phase is different with the exception of some overlapping. The pottery in the early phase is hand made of slow table turned whereas both hand made and wheel turned pottery appear in the upper levels. In the second phase i.e. from layer (15) some sherds of cord impressed ware, so characterstic of neolithic cultures in eastern India, were recovered. Some fine specimen of red burnished ware and chocolate coloured ware were also found from the middle levels along with some doubtful sherds of black and red ware. From the middle levels also some hand made sherds of red ware were recovered which had post firing paintings in red ocher. Among the common shapes met with were dishes bowls, vases, vases with carination at the waste and lids.

No metal was found during excavation but three pieces of polished stone tools (one an adze, one unfinished and one portion of the top of a stone celt were found (Pl. XXVII).

The important discovery was a good number of bone tools both of crude and finer variety. The tools were made from the bones (Pl. XXVI) of humped cattle, sheep/goat and antlers. In some cases semi-fossilised bones were used and flaking and pressure flaking techniques, reminiscent of late stone age, were current. The tool types showed points, burins, scrapers, digging tools, and the most important and interesting find was a single row harpoon made from antler bone. One other interesting find was a fragment of a blade on mineralised bone.

Besides the bone tools other bones recovered from excavations were of Elephus Maximus, Bovidae and Capra Hiccus Acgagisus.

The discovery of bone tools, provides a new horizon in the Proto-historic cultures of Orissa in particular and of the whole coastal region of eastern India in general.

B.K. SINHA

Archaeological Survey of India,
Excavation Branch, Bhubaneshwar.

Khaparkhera: A Submergible Chalcolithic Site

Khaparkhera, in district Dhar, Madhya Pradesh a small village on the right bank of the River Narmada is under threat of submersion by the proposed gigantic Sardar Sarovar reservoir. Surprisingly a large ancient settlement located in this village jurisdiction has so far remained unnoticed by the archaeologists.

This ancient settlement (Lat. 22° 4′ 16"N, Long 74° 51′ 28" E) known to the villagers as 'Vanitkhera', lies exactly on the right bank of Narmad about 600 m southeast of present village Khaparkhera. The name of the village seems to have been derived from this ancient mound, since Khaparkhera literally means 'a settlement of pot-sherds'. There is a small stream flowing on north and west side of the mound almost touching it, finally joining the Narmada. This settlement covers an area of more than 45,000 sq. m. (300 m x 150m) with a cultural deposit of about 9 m. resting on recent Narmada alluvium. It is almost undisturbed except for a few erosional gullies and cultivation on the surface of the mound. Since the bed rock is exposed on the right bank near the site, it prevents bank erosion. Probably this was the reason which attracted man to settle over here.

The surface collection made from the site by the author in October 1990 include various ceramic types industry such as northern black polished, black-and-red and red slipped ware, legged querns, mullers, terra-cotta skin rubbers and ear studs, microliths etc. The surface investigation and artefact types clearly suggest that the antiquity of the settlement goes back to chalcolithic times and continued during early historic period. Burnt bricks noticed at the site measure 25x20x8 cm and 38x28x10 cm. There is a Hanuman image carved on stone in bas relief lying on the top of the mound.

Apart from this, remains of a temple located about 300 m west of the site on the bank of

Narmada has also been noticed. Here there is thick deposit of yellowish alluvium which contains microliths mostly made of chalcedony.

The potentiality of the site immediate cries for horizontal excavation to throw light on the chalcolithic and early historic cultural phases of Malwa region before the site gets inundated and lost for ever.

Archaeological Survey of India,
Prehistory Branch, Nagpur.

S.B. OTA

Excavations at Ladyura, Almora, U.P.

Ladyura village Lat. 30° 35′ N, Long 80° 35′ E, Distt. Almora is situated in between the two perennial steams, the Ganghli and the Rigda just above their confluence point, nearly 1.5 km. north of Dangoli on Almora-Baijnath Gwaldum-Karanprayag road. The entire village is located on terraces formed by these rivulets. At least four terraces could easily be noticed. In the terraced fields there are a large number of cists which were first noticed by Shri M.P. Joshi of Kumun University - buried under lateritic clay, the thickness of which varies from 1 m to 2m. depending on the undulating surface.

As it was difficult to dig in the fields, three cists that were partly exposed at their southern ends were taken up for excavation (Pl. XXVIII).

All here available cists have been erected inside pits cut into the shale bed-rock. They are oriented north-south lengthwise and vary in size. Most of the cists are having only one compartment but few with more than one compartment are also available. They are open in the south. They are simple rectangular structures made out of a number of dressed shale slabs. The southern ends is always open.

The cists were erected inside the grave pit cut into the shale bed rock. One of the 'U' shaped grave pit is 0.80m. deep, 1.90m. long and 0.80m. wide at the top and 0.55 m. wide at the bottom. The verticality upright orthostats made by fixing their lower edges (lengthwise) in the grooves (channels) that have been cut into the bed rock. The space between the upright ends and groove margins has been packed with stone chips. Normally the channels have been so cut that their width tallies with the thickness of uprights for facilitating easy insertion and erection of uprights. The grooves are not very deep. The uprights have been covered with capping stones that run throughout the length of the cist. The capstone is normally the biggest and projects laterally on all sides across the top edges of the orthostats. Normally the northern end of the cist has been blocked by a single upright. The lateral ends of the rear (northern) orthostat would, almost invariably, never project out of the edges of the side orthostats, but rest firmly on them. On the sides in this case two uprights each have been erected. The second capping stone of the southern end is missing. The cist is 1.84 m. in length, 0.53m. in width and 0.45 m. in height and has been filled with self same material obtained by cutting the pit. One of the cap stone recoverd is 1 m in length and 0.64m. in width.

The most interesting feature of these cist burials is the presence of post holes on both sides (eastern and western) of the grave pit. Two post holes (0.16m. and 0.13m. in diameter) one on the east and the other in the west of the cist were found during excavation They are located almost equidistant from the upright orthostats of their respective sides, one on the north-western end and the other on the south eastern end of the cist. There is every possibility that similar, atleast two post-holes might have been there one on the south-western and the other on the north-eastern sides of the cists. These postholes have also been sunk in the bed-rock. The presence of the post holes indicates that after internment of the mortal remains and other funerary objects and after filling the pit, a conical shade supported atleast by four uprights (two on each side) and one central beam was erected over the burial. This is a noticed novel feature a noticed for the first time.

Tiny fragments of human bones were recovered from one of the cists. Other cists yielded fragments of iorn objects of indeterminate shape. This is due to highly corrosive and acidic nature of the overlying lateritic deposit and excessive rainfall.

POTTERY:

Cist No. 1

(1) Mostly coarse red ware, and with thick section, wheel made, ill fired. Mat impressions on the outer

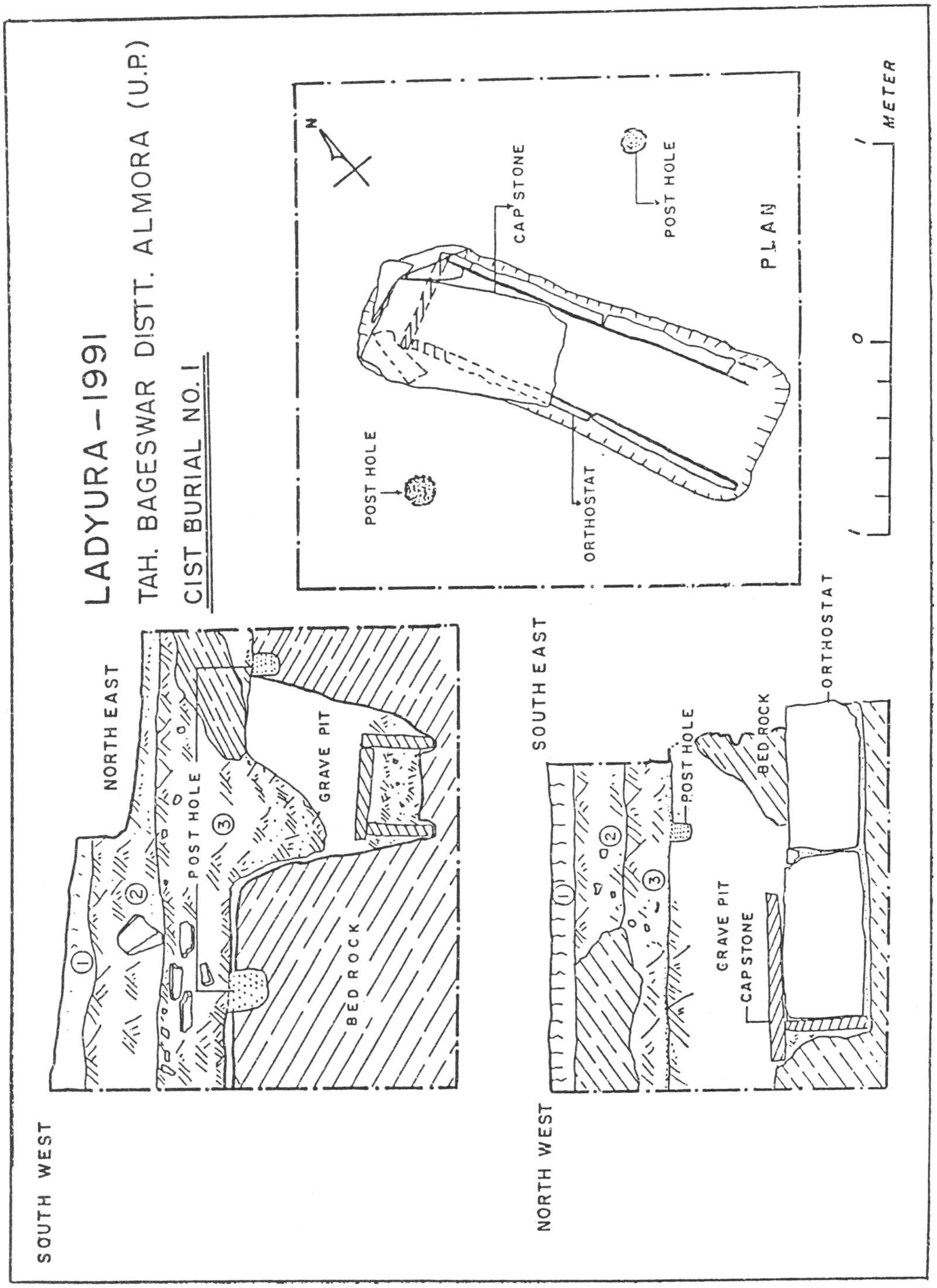

LADYURA-1991
TAH. BAGESWAR DISTT. ALMORA (U.P.)
CIST BURIAL NO. 1
N
CAP STONE
POST HOLE
PLAN
POST HOLE
ORTHOSTAT
0
1
METER
SOUTH WEST
NORTH EAST
1
2
3
POST HOLE
GRAVE PIT
BED ROCK
NORTH WEST
SOUTH EAST
ORTHOSTAT
BED ROCK
POST HOLE
GRAVE PIT
CAP STONE

surface. In few cases red slip is noticed on the outer surface.

(2) Grey ware, medium fabric, and with thick section. Wheel made, repared out of partially levigated clay and fired in reduction condition.

Cist No. 2

Black ware bowl with featureless rim, convex sides, thin section and of fine fabric. Wheel made, prepared out of well levigated clay and fired in reduction condition.

On the basis of the pottery recovered from these burials, they could be dated to around first or second century B.C. This is tentative till the results of TL dating are available.

Fortunately in the area of Koormand and Bechandhar, which are located near the confluence of Ram ganga and Kauravagand rivers, on the right bank of the former and on the left bank of the later a number of cist burials are located. Grave pits for these cists have been cut into the last aggredational deposits of the two rivers and have been filled with the self same material. At Bechandhar right over the filling of the grave pits and also over the last aggredational deposit there is a later habitational deposit of nearly 1 m. yielding fine red wares very similar to Kushan pottery. This evidence also corroborates the date as above.

Archaeological Survey of India,
Prehistory Branch, Nagpur.

A.K. SHARMA

Harappan Horned Deity: The Evidence from Padri in Western India

Three intact painted storage jars were recovered from the rural Harappan site at Padri in Talaja taluk of Bhavnagar district, Gujarat. Two of them decorated with the horned deity motif. The village Padri Gohil ni lies roughly 50 km south of Bhavnagar town and 8 km west of Talaja. A small excavation here, carried out by the Department of Archaeology, Deccan College, Post-Graduate and Research Institute, Pune in 1990-91, has yielded very promising results. Some new features like rectangular mud structures similar to those unearthed in the chalcolithic levels in Deccan and a new painted ceramic, which is coarse in fabric, have come to light. The ancient habitation, 2.5 km south of the present village, is locally known as *kerala-ne-Dhoro,* meaning, according to the local inhabitants, the habitat of the fishing tribe called "kera".

These intact and unusually large painted storage jars were taken out by the villages while digging the site for earth to construct houses. However, we could identify their exact find spots. Of the three jars, two are in sturdy red ware and one in buff. The largest jar of sturdy red ware, only of its kind found so far, is 81 cm high with a circumference of 2.34m. It is decorated with a linear human figure wearing a horned headgear. The other jar in buff ware bears three motifs of a horned headgear.

Horned human figures and headgears were earlier reported from such sites as Kalibangan (Rajasthan State), Mohenjo-daro and Kot Diji (Western Pakistan), but for the fist time Gujarat has produced significant evidence in this respect. The discovery of the motifs of horned deity suggest an early date for the Harappans at Padri, but the ceramic assemblage resembles that of Rojdi B, which has been dated to 2200-2000 B.C. (Possehl and Raval 1989: 171).

The painted designs include a panel (12 cm broad) of a light yellow organge colour bordered by a triple horizontal band which a human figure with a horned headgear (Pl. XXIX). The horns shown here look similar to those of the special species of bull, locally known as *kankrej,* found in Saurashtra and Kutch. Only the upper half of the figure is seen in the panel whereas the portion below the waist extends beyond over the red surface of the pot also. The head of the figure is represented by a small solid circle, to which is attached the prominent curved hatched horns, 14 cm in length. They touch the upper border of the panel. The braided hair, 7 cm long, is seen on the left-hand side of the figure. The torso and the hands are 8 cm long. The garment on the waist, resembling a grass skirt, extends to the knees (length 7 cm); it is represented by slanting wavy lines. The human figure is a male as the genitalia would suggest. The legs are solid and 9 cm long. The total height of the figure without horns is 18 cm and 25 cm with horns. The human figurine is flanked by two pairs of two curved lines on the right and three pairs on the left. They emanate from the group of three vertical wavy lines at the base of the motifs where two sets of curved lines join. The design, represented by three curved lines, ends with hatched curves, the tips of which bear three short strokes attached to solid circles.

The light yellow organge panel and the red surface below give an impression of land and water surfaces respectively. The human figure, therefore appears to be standing in water. The running loop like curved lines flanking the horned human figure are confined to the panel whereas the vertical wavy lines extend below it. They most probably represent some kind of water plant with their leaves and roots on land and in water respectively. The horned deity is shown moving forward with its right leg and hand brought forward and the left ones backward.

Similar figure, but in a seated posture and surrounded by four animals namely an elephant, a tiger, a rhinoceros and a buffalo, noticed on one of the Harappan seals (No 420) from Mohenjo-daro in Pakistan, has been identified as the prototype of the Hindu deity 'Siva' (Mackay 1938. Pl. XCIV). In Hindu mythology 'Siva' is described as seated in a yoga-like posture and a trident *(trishul)* as an emblem is always associated with him. The head-dress of the figure on the seal from Mohenjo-daro, composed of two horns and a tall central portion, is suggestive of the shape of trident. The group of animals around this figure evokes Siva's later aspect as *pasupati,* "Lord of Beasts" (Srinivasan 1975-76). During Caspers (1989), however, questions this identification in view of its much lesser frequency of depiciton. A human figure wearing a horned headgear incised on a terracotta cake at Kalibangan (Rajasthan state) (Lal 1979) looks more identical with the Padri motif because both of them are shown standing. The painted motif from Padri is very significant and could be associated with the religious beliefs of the Harappans in Saurashtra. The horned deity on this jar could be identified as that of a *pasupati,* the lord of the beasts as it is surrounded by a natural scene such as vegetation.

During Caspers (1989) is of the opinion that these horned human figurines signify the existence of an ancient hunting cult with rites and practices which may have become blurred with the passing time. She further states that they may well mark the presence of a minority group of basically non-Harappan inhabitants whose original home has to be sought in one of the regions to the north of Greater Indus Plains, such as present-day Afghanistan, the Kashmir region or western Nepal. This explanation is hard to accept because the evidence from various Harappan sites points to the existence of a very strong system of state organization, one of the characteristic features of which is the presence of a priestly class and religious ideology. The sporadic occurrence of idols or motifs of religious importance, could be attributed to the possibility that the right of making and possessing such objects of religious importance was available only to the people of very high social ranking in the society. With the discovery of a horned headed figure in Gujarat, there is hardly any doubt that the worship of this deity was prevalent almost all over the Harappan state. To what extent certain customs or traditions of a small local tribe would have influenced the civilized and urbanite Harappans, spread over a very vast territory, is a matter of debate. Had the hunting cult been prevlent among any local tribe in Sind, its influence would not have been felt in far off places like Rajasthan or Gujarat.

The other jar in the Buff ware (Trench OX3), 72.5 cm high and having the circumference of 1.86 m, bears, on its upper part, three decorative motifs of a horned headgear with loose hair, represented by six vertical wavy lines emanating from the bottom part of it (Pl. XXX). They are bordered by a double horizontal band. The large curved and hatched horns are attached to a roughly squarish headgear, measuring 5 cm x 4.5 cm. The width between two horns varies from 16 cm to 21 cm. Some of the wavy lines representing the hair extend even beyond the lower bordering double band. Of the three motifs, the horns of two end with solid circles and one with sharp points. This motif is also new and could have represented "pasupati" in different form.

Two parallels, e.g. a horned-headed deity in gold in Hissar IIIc (Iran) and a painting on a pot at Kot Diji (Western Pakistan) deserve special mention in this connection. At Hissar IIIc five gold sheets with a mouflon (wild mountain sheep of souther Europe) or ibex were found in a hoard. The horned sheets bore seven pairs of perforations, which pierced the long coiled horns and the beard of the animal (Schmidt 1937: 189. fig. 111. pl. XLVI). A pot at Kot Diji bore the gracefully curved horns painted in black with a six petaled flower within them. From the junction of the horns seems to hang down an elongated human head, its chin and cheeks shown in black dots, the lower forehead and the upper part of the long drooping ears in solid black (Khan 1965: 57. fig. 16. pl. XVIIb). The difference between the

Padri and Kot Diji motifs is that the former is depicted with curly long hair whereas the latter is represented by an elongated human head. Sankalia (1969) feels the origin of this motif took place in Iran, but on reaching Sind, it was humanized and the mouflon horns were replaced by those of a bull. A similar horned (bucranian) motif decorated on Red ware pot has been reported from the Neolithic site of Burzahom in Kashmir (Kaw 1979). The occurrence of this motif, out side the Harappan domain, is significant and points to the cultural contact with its contemporaries, the Neolithic culture.

VASANT SHINDE

Department of Archaeology,
Deccan College Post-graduate Research Institute,
Pune.

REFERENCES

During Caspers, E.C.L. 1989. Magic hunting practices in Harappan times in Karen Frefeit and Per Sorensen (eds.) *South Asian Archaeology*. 1985. Copenhagen: 227-236. Scandinavian Institute of Asian Studies.Sankalia, H.D. 1969. Kot Diji and Hissar III. *Antiquity*. 43: 142-44.

Kaw, R.N. 1979. The Neolithic culture of Kashmir. in D.P. Agrawal and D.K. Chakrabarti (eds.) *Essay in Indian Protohistory* New Delhi: 219-228.

Khan, F.A. 1965. Excavations at Kot Diji *Pakistan Archaeology*. 2: 13-85.

Lal, B.B. 1979. Kalibangan and Indus Civilization. in D.P. Agrawal and D.K. Chakrabarti (eds.) *Essays in Indian Protohistory* New Delhi. 65-97.

Mackay, E.J.H. 1938. *Further Excavations at Mohenjo-daro*. 2. Delhi: Government of India Press.

Possehl, Gregory L. and M.H. Raval 1989. *Harappan Civilization and Rojdi*. New Delhi.

Schmidt, E.F. 1937. *Excavations at Tepe Hissar, Damghan*. Philadelphia. Pennsylvania University.

Srinivasan, D. 1975-76. The so-called Proto-Siva seal from Mohenjo-daro: An iconological assesment. *Archives of Asian Art*. XXIX: 47-58.

Identification of Pundravardhana

On the western bank of the dried - up bed of the River Mahanand, and situated at a distance of 104 km to the north -west of Malda Town and 2 km to the north of Samsi railway station on the Howrah/Sealdah - Silliguri section of the Eastern Railway is one of the largest sites in the country, measuring approx. 7.5 km 0.75km, the longer axis being from north to south. Three villages, viz. Sanjip, Domanabheda and Kandaran, have encroached upon the mound out of which Kandaran seems to be the oldest settlement at the site. The railway track has cut across the mound at its southern extremity in such a way that a strip of about 0.5 km of the mound lies to the south of this track.

The land around the mound is subjected to cultivation which has destroyed much of the evidence of this ancient settlement. Still, at places, particularly towards the western and the southern end, traces of rampart and moat can be seen.

The exploration (IAR 1980-81) has revealed sherds of Black Polished Ware, Northern Black Polished Ware, stamped pottery of the Kushana-Gupta tradition, red ware and black ware of the mediaeval period and glazed ware. The main shape in the N.B.P. Ware, is bowls and dishes of coarser fabric The same types are also met within the black-slipped ware. Among the shapes of the red ware mention may be made of bowls with incurved rim, dishes and vases, Few tiles have also been found. At places the remains the brick structure were also noticed. On the basis of the ceramic tradition the antiquity of the site can safely be dated to the sixth-fifth century B.C.

Among other finds, mention may be made of terracotta figurines datable to the second third cent by A.D. One of these figurines is a horse with somewhat elongated neck with incised design indicating the mane. Another broken female figurine having hair tied at the top of the head in the shape of a bun has long eyes and big round ear-rings. Both these figurines are moulded, made of well lavigated clay and are well burnt. These pieces are now kept in the Malda Museum.

Two stone sculptures, kept in the said museum belong to this site. The first sculpture in black stone is unfinished and shows very clear chisel marks. This standing sculpture represents Bṛihaspati, carrying the *śruka* (?) and *kamaṇḍalu* (Bhattacharya: 8. pl. IV 1). Another sculpture is that of Vishṇu, again in the stone, which is broken from the waist. Both these figures are the work of the Pala-Sena artists.

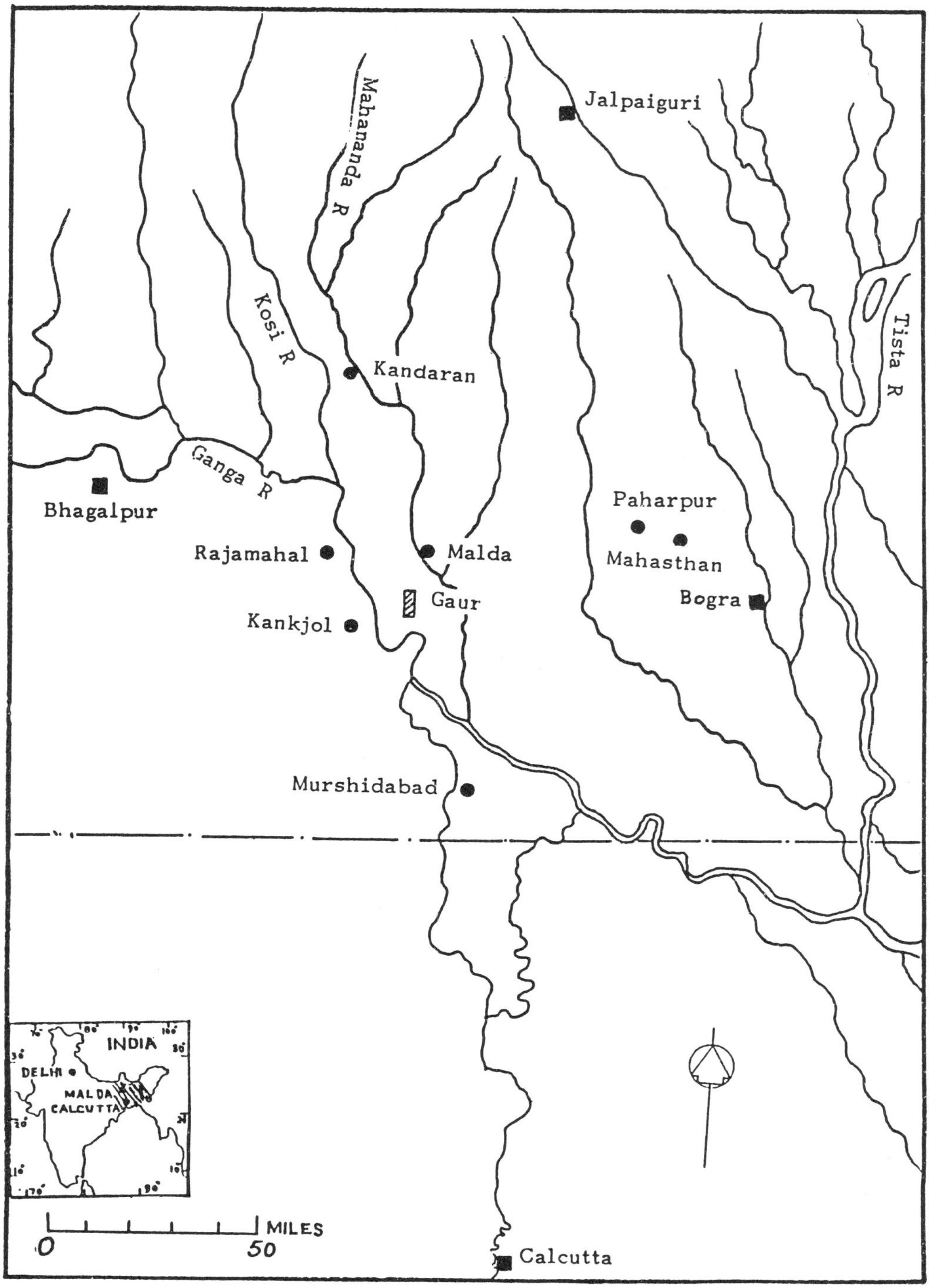

Fig.1. Map showing Kandaran (Dist. Malda, West Bengal) and other ancient sites.

General A. Cunninghum has not mentioned this site in his 'Report'. The earliest mention of this site, as 'medieval mound' is made by A.K Maitreya (p. 24) but he does not give any further description of the site.

This site is part of Varindra or Varendra also known as Pundra Desa or Puṇḍravardhana as both the districts of Malda and West Dinajpur of West Bengal were once, part of Puṇḍravardhana. The very name of Kandaran, one of the three villages situated on the mound, does remind us of a city called Puṇḍravardhana. But this ancient city has, already, been identified with the present site of Mahasthangarh, Dist. Bogra (Bangla Desh) (ASIR XV) by other later scholars. Therefore, in the light of the literary and other records we will have to probe the problem of the proper identification of Pundravardhana afresh.

Chakraborty, on the basis of the description of the *Mahābhārata,* describes the Puṇḍra as living in the tract between Aṅga and the Kauśikī marshes. To the north of them were the Kirātas and to their south-east were the Vaṅgas. The Suṁhas and the Tāmraliptikas were living towards the south-east of their territory (JASB IV). Beyond doubt, Chakraborty had deduced his conclusion from the epic, which, while describing the exploit of Bhīma, the third Pāṇḍava, mentions that after conquering Anga, he subdued Pauṇḍra-Vāsudeva, the powerful king of Kauśikīkachchha. Then after conquering Samudrasena and Chandrasena, the kings of Tamralipti and Karvat, he subdued the Suṁhas on the sea-coast (27.19-23). From the above description it is clear that the River Kauśikī (modern Kosi) must have been very close to the Puṇḍra's territory. It is pertinent to mention here that the epic does not mention the River Kārātoya, on the bank of which Mahasthangarh is situated. Had Bhīma defeated the Puṇḍra king whose capital was on the bank of the Kārātoya, instead of the Kauśikī the name of the former would have been used. But this is not the case and surprisingly from Kandaran one of the branch of the Kauśikī or Kosi is only 19 km (Buchavan 1986). The River Kosi is notorious for changing its course, and it is not surprising that during the epic age it would have been near the mound.

Hieun - Tsang has described Pundravardhana to be 600 li (160 km.) from Kājingara or Kājangala (modern Kankajol). Kankajol is approx. 25 km. south of Rajamahal and about the same distance to the south-west of Gauda (Malda Dist.). From Gauda to Malda is 24 km. and from there Kandaran is situated at a distance of about 104 km. If we add all these distances it will come to 153 km. which is almost the same as mentioned by the Chinese pilgrim as the distance of Puṇḍravardhana from Kajangala. On the basis of this presumption we can safely conclude Kandaran to be the site of Puṇḍravardhana. The other site, Mahasthanagarh, is approx. 158 km. from Kankajol, but this distance is on the basis of 'as crow files' and not based upon the exact land route, which must be more than 160 km.

Hieun-Tsang mentions the city of Puṇḍravardhana to be of about 30 li around (5 miles or 8 km. in circumference). As mentioned earlier the circumference of Kandaran site is around 16.50 km. where the mound of Mahasthanagarh is only 15000 feet in circumference (Beal 1958), which does not tally with the description of the city of Pundravardhana as described by the Chinese traveller. The mound of Kandaran exactly fits in the description.

It is generally believed that since the famous Mahasthanagarh inscription of the third cent. B.C., which refers to Puṇḍravardhana, was discovered from this site (Mahasthanagarh), it represents the ancient city - Puḍravardhana, but even a cursory reading of the said inscription will show that the inscription mentions not only the name of Puṇḍravardhana but also mentions the names of the Suṁhas and Sulakshmī, (XXI). Thus, on the basis of this inscription also we cannot say that the present site of Mahasthanagarh represents Puṇḍravardhana.

No ancient writer has mentioned Mahasthanagarh as either Puṇḍravardhana or as the capital of the Puṇḍras. In the *Rāmacharita* also, Sandhyakara Nandī (contemporary of Kumārapāla, 11th century A.D.) does not mention Mahasthanagarh though it does mention Vārendra and Puṇḍravardhana. In fact, it is only the *Kārātoya Mahātmya* cent A.D.) which describes Puṇḍravardhana on the bank of the Karatoya. This may be due to the reason that on account of the Muslim onslaught the Hindu rulers shifted their capital from the present site of Kandaran to Mahasthanagarh, another important Puṇḍra city. It is, only after this later event that Mahasthanagarh gained importanance and the contemporary writers started eulogising this place as the Pundra capital.

The above discussion leads to ascertain that the modern village Kandaran is the site of ancient Pundravardhana.

Archaeological Survey of India,
Janpath, New Delhi.

ACHYUTANAND JHA

REFERENCES

Archaeological Survey of India Report. Delhi 1969 XV: 37
Beal, S. 1958. Buddhist Records of the Western World (Travels of Hieun Tsang). Calcutta. IV: 403-4.
Bhattacharya, M. Art In stone. *Catalogue of Sculptures in Malda Museum.* Calcutta.
Buchanan, Francis. 1986 (reprint). An Account of The District of Purnea In 1809-10, Delhi: 23-28.
Chakraborty, Manmohan. Notes on the geography of Old Bengal. *Journal of the Asiatic Society of Bengal* IV. 5: 268-9.
Epigrphia Indica XXI: 85.
Indian Archaeology 1980-81 A Review: 77.
The Mahabharata Sabhaparvan 27. 19-23.
Maitreya, A.K. The Ancient Monuments of Varendra: 24.

Discovery of an early Inscription from Pitalkhora

The rock-cut caves of Pitalkhora (LAT. 20°20'N, Long. 75° 00' E) well known Hīnayāna Buddhist complex, came into view about the year 1851 (Wilson 1853), wherein a brief description of the main chaitya cave (cave No. 3) and the adjoining Vihāra (cave No. 4) was highlighted. Subsequently, Jas Burgess (1883) drew the attention of scholars to the inscriptions from these caves recording donations of individuals towards the excavations of these caves and other welfare measures.The donors among others are devotees from Patiṭhāna (Pratishṭhāna) or modern Paiṭhan in Maharashtra.

M.G. Dikshit (1941) worked on these caves and discovered a couple of them on the south of the ravine. But, it was M.N. Deshpande (1959) who for the first time published a detailed study on these caves. He has added four more inscriptions to the existing list.

In a recent field work at Pitalkhora, I have come to another inscription (Pl. XXXI) recorded in cave No. 4 over a pilaster (On the left side) to right of the cave. It consists of six letters of early Brāhmī Character and in Prākrit language. It reads *Bhāta Rakhitāya*, i.e. brother of Rakshita or monk Rakshita. The inscription is seemingly incomplete. The upper stroke of each letter falls almost in one horizontal line, though there is no uniformity in the lower part of the characters in their finish. The inscription is datable to a period between 250-200 B.C., on the basis of charts drawn by Vidya Dehejia (1972), S. Nagaraju (1981) and Ojha (1975). The letters are analysed on these lines. A close examination of these letters reveals that the letter *'bha'* has a typical vertical stroke of Mauryan character and slightly drooping left stroke with an unconventionally placed medial sign of ā attached to it (the medial sign is placed like in the case of letter *dha, ba* and *tha.* instead of at the top end of the vertical stroke. Its similarity can be noticed at Girnār, Sāñchi, and Bhājā. The letter *ta* with a vertical stroke emerging out of inverted English capital letter *'V'*. In the case of second the medial sign is attached to the usual top almost at right angle, a feature normally coinciding with Aśokan Brāhmī. Its similarity can be noticed at Bharhut, Girnar, Sanchi, Ghosundi. Similarly letter *'ra'* too has Mauryan affinity and is comparable with Girnār, Bhārhut, Sāñchi etc. The letter *'kha'* like the above three letters has close similarity with the early Indian Brāhmī script. Similar *'kha'* can be seen at Sañchi, Sopara, Girnar, Amravati. The sixth letter *'Ya'* has a typical Mauryan boat shaped lower stroke attached to the central vertical stroke and in this representation all the three ends of the letter are almost on one horizontal line which is seldom seen in early Brāhmī alphabets. However, it denotes an early character of Bhāhmī script with its close similarity noticed at Besnagar, Ghosundi, Bharhut, Sanchi, Gaya, Bhaja, Karla and Junnar etc. Rakshita of the inscription deys exact identity. However such name occurs in ceylonese Buddhist chronicle Mahāvaṁsa (1912) in connection with Buddhist missionaries who were despatched by Aśoka to different parts of his realm and the adjacent countries for propagation of Buddhist doctrine, after the conclusion of third Buddhist council held at Pāṭaliputra. Geiger Wilhelm (1912. VI) and Mookerji (1955). assign the date of the third Buddhist council to 247 B.C. and 253 B.C. respectively, while some scholars assign the same to 250 B.C. by taking into account the date of birth of Lord Buddha as 566 B.C.

According to Mahāvaṁsa the following Rakshitas were deputed as missionries to the deccan.

1)	Rakshita	Vanavāsi	Present Banavāsc
2)	Yona Dharmarakkhita (possibly a Greek Monk)	Aparāntaka	Northern half of Bombay coast

3) Mahādharma Rakshita	Marāṭhā country	Possibly present Marathwada region.

Apart from this, there is epigraphical evidence of Rakshita in a Vihāra at Pandulena caves, near Nasik, Maharashtra (Senart 1905-06). Here Rakshita occurs as a donor along with his father.

The newly discovered inscription thus corroborates the literary evidence provided in Mahāvaṁsa.*

Archaeological Survey of India,
Aurangabad Circle,
Aurangabad.

S.K. MITRA

REFERENCE

Burgess, Jas. 1883. Report on the Buddhist Cave Temples and their Inscriptions. *Arch. Surv. West. Ind. IV. London:* 11-12.

Dehejia, Vidya. 1972. *Early Buddhist Rock Temples. Thames and Hudson. London.* Tables 1-2 and 4-5.

Deshpande, M.N. 1959. The Rock-cut caves of Pitalkhora in the Deccan, *Ancient India.* 15. New Delhi: 66-93.

Dikshit, M.G. 1941. Fresh light on the Pitalkhora caves. *Jour. Bombay Historical Soc. 1-2:* 112-21.

Mookerji, Radha Kumud. 1955. *Asoka.* Delhi: 46.

Nagaraju, S. 1981. *Buddhist Architecture of Western India, Delhi.* Chart II.

Ojha, G.S. 1975. Bharatiya Prachin Lipimala. New Delhi: Lipipatra I.

Senart, E. 1905-06. The Inscriptions in the caves at Nasik. *Epigraphia Indica. VIII-E. Hultzsch Ed. Calcutta:* pl. V (N.3).

Wilhelm Geiger. 1912. *The* Mahāvaṁsa. London: 82 ff.

Wilson, J. 1853. *Jour. Bombay Br. Roy. As. Soc. IV:* 357-60.

Role of Temples in Medieval Orissa

Medieval Orissa witnessed the construction of a number of temples. Though the primary role of these high edifices was religion but gradually and simultaneously their role became multidimensional. Their contribution to the fields of art, architecture, society, economy, polity and above all to the culture of Orissa is quite immense. Though the temples in other parts of India played such roles, there is some speciality in case of Orissan temples because of the circumstances leading to the building of these temples. Here geographical and physical aspects of Orissa proper played parts. Then various political forces vied with each other to build lasting testimonials to their grandeur and power. They became artistic mainstay of the Orissan people their to keep alive the traditional and cultural fabric of their society in the midst of constantly changing political scene. As a result the Odissi dance, music, drama and moral outlook, social phenomenon, creative desires, artistic activities have their direct link to the existing temples. The artistically rich temples have kept the traditions and the artistic glory alive since the earliest times. As a result the artistic class from generation to generation experimented the artistic designs on stone and reached the climax in the 13th century in the Sun Temple at Konarak.

During the Sailodbhavas, Bhaumakaras, Somavamsis and the Gangas numerous temples were built and art and artistic activities flourished to a great extent. The religious convictions of Orissan people have made its cultural heritage rich and sound.

Orissa was the only region which retained the great religions like Jainism, Buddhism, Saivism and Vaisnavism for a long period than any other region of India. Long after Jainism and Buddhism lost their hold at their original places of prominence they were seen thriving in Orissa with much of their pristine glory. Saivism also saw its popularity as Bhubaneswar became the Sivakhetra and came to be known as Kasi of the east Vaisnavism is still centered in Orissa with the cult of Jagannatha as supreme (Misra 1971). The creativity of the people was an important factor for cultural enrichment. From the time of Asoka's Dhauli and Kharavela's Kumari complex to the time of Konark, it was a long experiment in the artistic line through generations. Their exploration on thought, cult, imagination lead to the conclusion that sculptural art was almost prevalent as hereditary profession of the people. The Socioeconomic stability was a vital factor for the cultural growth of Orissa.

The valleys of Orissa were productive and fertile, the self sufficiency of the people. Maritime trade was

* On palaeographical grounds the insciption seems to belong to the latter half of the 2nd century B.C. or first half of the first century B.C. which also corresponds to the date of the cave and it can be read as '*Bhūtarakbhtāya*' (=*for Bhūtarakshita*) - B.R. Mani.

flourishing; as a result the economy of the State was in sound footing. This helped the rulers to start their building activities at considerable public expenditure.

The social customs, caremonies, rites and rituals paved the way for the growth of art, music, drama, dances and craft all in their traditional form. Many years might have elapsed and many political convulsions have come and gone but the great caremonies like car festivals and *Boita Bandhana* did not change its traditional character. Similarly time has not obliterated folk art, village crafts and stone carvings even today which are the mainstay of many people of Orissa. According to the *Shilpa Prakash* (a manuscript on temple building) the patron of the temple will always have peace, wealth, grain and sons. The erection of a temple for the Gods was undertaken for the benefit of the whole community whose spiritual aspiration it embodied (Michell 1977).

A temple is not the house of a priest or an ascetic. It is the physical core as well as the soul of the community. It is meant to instruct man in the greatness of his race and elevate his soul in the pursuit of God. Every temple in India is a definite architectural piece and sculptural treasure house. The sculptures depict the story of the race; in the words of Coomarswami, "the Indian temple is the statement of a racial experience and serves the purpose of life, like daily bread Coomarswami 1927).

In the Kalinga style of temples, besides the role of the *Jagamohana* as the assembly hall for the devotees, the *natamandir* played the role of entertaining the God by the *devadasis* or dancing girls. The *bhogamandapa* is meant for the offering of the *bhoga* to god. The Bhubaneswar inscription of the Ganga King Anangabhimadeva III(El XXX) mentions that the *Mandapa* was used for performing festivals on auspicious occasions. *Mahotsavas* and ceremonies were also allowed to be performed. The dancing girls who were meant for entertaining the God were granted Land by the king. The origin of the custom may be traced to the need of Gods at the time of god's worship and popular festivals. The priests recited the vedas and *puranas* in the temple (EI XXVIII).

The Medieval Hindu temple is a state with in the State with its own administration, finance, employees and traditions. Next to the state itself, it was the biggest employer, the great patron of art, culture and learning. It was the centre of higher education which attracted the best talent both among the teacher and the taught and it was the greatest centre of entertainment for the commonman.

Music is the language through which our inexpressible thoughts and feelings find expression. Hence it is a superb and divine art. If we go to the earliest inscriptional evidence, we find in the Hathi Gumpha inscription references to vocal and instrumental music, dance and drama in ancient Kalinga. The great monuments like Lingaraga and Konark depict various instruments for music and dance poses. There is a continuity of musical traditions in Orissa. (Sahu 1956). The dance poses are remarkable at Konark from where the Odissi dance has taken birth. The *devadasi* system in which the dancing girls were dedicated to Gods attached to temples earlier prevailed in Kashmir, Bengal, Saurashtra, Rajasthan, Andhra, Maharashtra, Karnataka, Tamilnadu and Orissa. In Orissa the system is still prevalent.

In Medieval times Oriya poets wrote their ornamental *Kavya* keeping in mind the pattern of Orissan temples. To them each *Kavya* was like a temple, architecturally solid covered thickly with imagery like the sculptures from start to finish (Mana sing 1962).

The credit for such goes to Anangabhimadeva III (1211-1238) who employed 36 orders and 97 classes for the service of God Jagannath (Sahu 1956).

The Orissan temples played significant and dynamic role not only in the sphere of culture but also became a repository of the traditions of society and religion. It became not only a religious place but also a learning center, a theater, a debating place, and a place of unity and solidarity of the masses and harbinger of peace and tranquillity during the Medieval period.

Archaeological Survey of India,
Janpath, New Delhi.

K.P. PADHY

REFERENCES

Coomaraswamy, A.K. 1927. *Introduction to Indian Art.* Madras: VI

Das, M.N. (ed.) 1978. *Sidelights on History and Culture of Orissa.* Cuttack: I

Epigraphia India. XXVII. New Delhi. 1949-50: 334; XXX. New Delhi. 1953-54: 23.

ManSingh, M. 1962. *History of Oriya Literature.* New Delhi: 3.

Michell, George. 1977. *The Hindu Temple.* London: 38.

Misra, K.C. 1971. The cult of Jagannath. Calcutta: 43.

Sahu, N.K. (ed.) 1956a. *A History of Orissa.* Calcutta I: 127-28.

Sahu, N.K. (ed.) 1956b. *A History of Orissa.* Calcutta II: 397-404.

The Northern Black Polished and Other Associated Wares from Ropar

The mound of Ropar, renamed Rupnagar (30^{0} 58′ N. Lat; 76° 32′ E. Long) district rupnagar (erstwhile in Dt. Ambala) is located left bank of Satluj. It is a 21 m high mound and was excavated between 1952 and 1955 by the Archaeological Survey of India under the direction of Y.D. Sharma (Sharma 1956). The excavations unfolded a sequence of six cultural periods. to recapitulate, the periods from bottom upwards are; Period I, Harappa (C. 2100 to 1400 B.C.); Period II. Painted Grey Ware (C. 1000 to 600 B.C.); Period III, Norther Black Polished ware or early historical (C. 600 to 200 B.C.); Period IV, middle to late historical (C. 200 B.C. to 700 A.D.); Period V, late Historical (C. 700 - 1200); and Period VI, Medieval (C. 1200 -1700). Of these Period III, yielded the Northern Black Polished ware (hereafter NBPW). Before getting into the details of pottery, a word about the salient features of this period may not be out of place.

The Period III at Ropar, which covers a time-span of about four hundred years, and definable in terms of introduction and disappearance of NBPW, has further been divided into two sub-Periods - A and B - on the basis of structural and pottery evidences. The significant point about this period is that it has yielded over four-hundred and fifty NBPW sherds despite limited area of excavation. Out of these nearly 85 sherds come from sub-Period III A alone. The large presence of these sherds at Ropar is in striking contrast to other sites of comparable date away from the epicentre of the NBPW which supposed to be in the mid-Ganga Valley. Sharma is of the opinion that NBPW arrived at Ropar through pilgrims and traders, although it is likely that this *delux* ware at Ropar later began to be manufactured locally. That NBPW at Ropar later began to be manufactured locally. That NBPW at Ropar was prized commodity is proved by some broken NBP pots whose were carefully rivetted together with copper wire pieces through rivet holes. The evidence is important but difficult to substanstiate whether it implies the ware's economical or ritual significance or both.

Largely, the NBPW sherds at Ropar are monochrome covering that shades of jet-black, steel-blue and somewhat grayish occasionally showing reddish-brown speckles on the surface. Position of bichrome sherds at Ropar is doubtful. A good number of sherds of sherds have a fine body fabric and hard to scrap. They bear glossy surface slip with lustrous seen. Some of the sherds in the collection are as fine as the top-graded NBPW. In general, the core of the NBPW sherds is mostly red, but in some cases, grayish core have also been met with. In a few instances, the NBPW slip on sherds has peeled off resulting in exposing the red matt surface and grayish core.

On the whole, the NBPW at Ropar does not form a homogeneous mass probably precluding production of NBP pots out of a single firing technique. The technical investigations carried out on NBPW vessels now hold, albeit not yet free from doubt, that there was no standard technique to produce NBPW pots. The investigations further maintain that the heterogeneous slip appearing as glossy metallic sheen on the NBPW pot is resultant of such factors as firing conditions (oxidizing and reducing), the fineness of slip (termed as *Kabiz,* which is largely a preparation of natural ingredients) and the iron oxide added to it, and the range of temperature applied while baking (Sahay 1969: 146).

As the date of the NBPW period at Ropar, it is pertinent to recall here that the time beacket of 6th-4th B.C. assigned by Sharma has not been accepted by Sinha (1969). Sinha is of the view that spread of the NBPW actually took place in at least two widely differing contexts - primary (early) and the other, secondary (late). The primary context, according to him, lies in the mid Ganga Valley comprising parts of eastern Uttar Pradesh and Western Bihar, represented at sites like Rajghat, Kausambi, Sravasti, Rajgir, Vaisali and Taxila, and the secondary, at Hastinapur,, Ropar, Ujjain, Navdatoli, Charsada, etc.

Thus according to this hypothesis, Sinha includes Ropar under the NBPW sites of secondary distribution and further argues that the NBPW at Ropar cannot be dated earlier than the 4th century B.C. In support of his point of view Sinha, among other things, also takes note of an incribed sealing of an early Mauryan date in addition to the moulded terracotta human figurines of about 3rd Century B.C., which were found from the NBPW levels. It has been observed that the NBPW yielding layers at Ropar were not very much below those levels from where the sealing and terra-cotta human figurines were recovered (Sinha 1969).

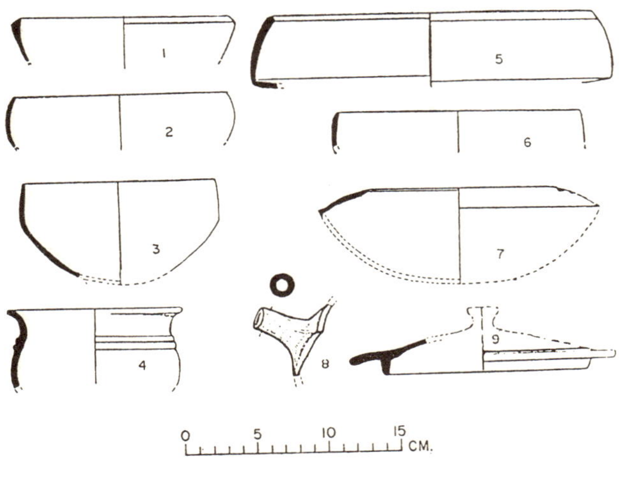

Fig. 1. Ropar: NBP ware from Period III

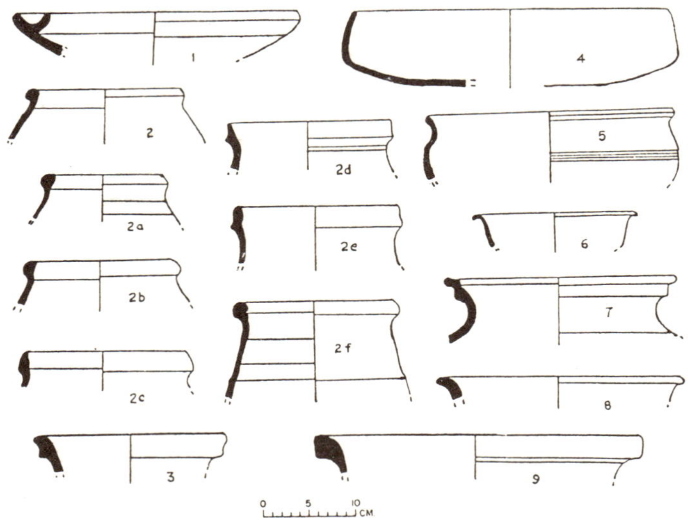

Fig. 2. Ropar: Red ware from Period II

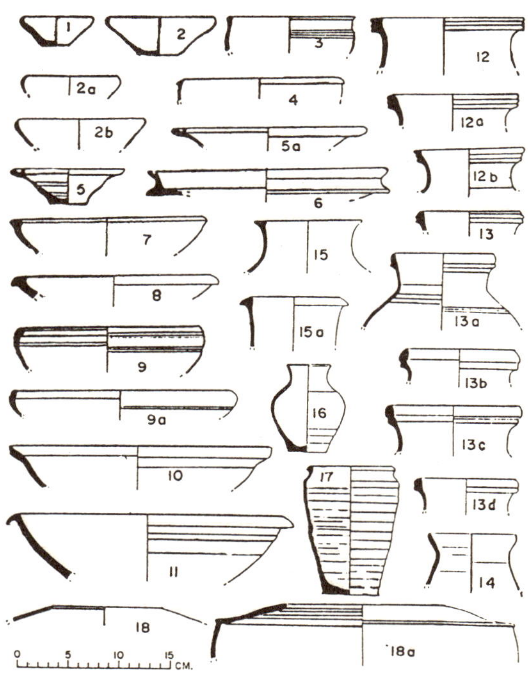

Fig. 3. Ropar: Red ware from sub-Period

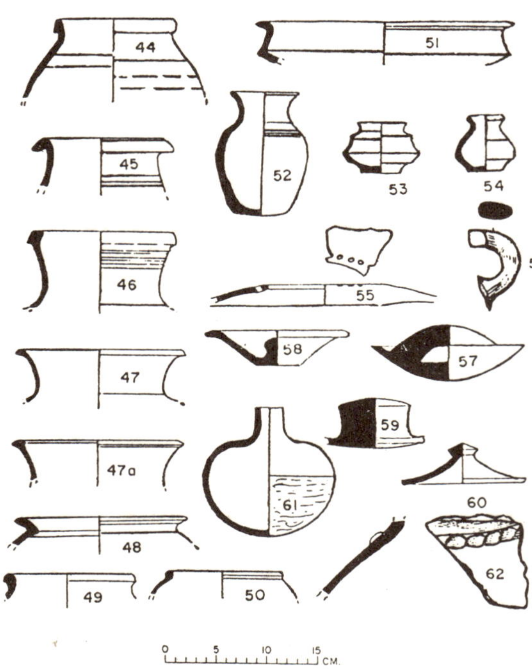

Fig. 4. Red ware from sub-Period III B

Despite all these arguments, the NBPW date at Ropar does not seem to have finally been settled. It is felt that the NBPW period at Ropar, like Taxila, has adequate evidences to have witnessed a developed, prosperous phase of urban character right from the beginning of the early historical period. The period in question clearly documents sanitary contrivances in the form of ring lined soaked wells occurring in clusters and singly remains of lapidary workshop, impressive architectural remains as evidenced by a 3.65 m. wide and 75 m. long retaining wall of kiln-burnt bricks, stamps and objects of skilled craftsmanship, implements of copper and iron, carved stone objects, proofs of literacy in the form of sealings, copper bear coins, punched marked coins of copper and silver with silver cast coins, etc., all pointing towards a well established town life. Such a cultural advancement naturally presupposes active trade links with other sites and a sort of conducive background which may have built up over some long periods of time. What we feel is that unless a total analysis of the NBPW complex of Ropar in relation to actual conditions viz. socioeconomic, religious, and if possible, political - prevailing at the time of its emergence at Ropar is attempted, the question of dating of this diagnotic ware at least at Ropar will remain only tentative.

The principal shapes of the NBPW reported from Ropar include; bowls (both shallow and deep), dishes vases or *handi* spouted vessels and lids (Fig. 1).

The other associated wares with the NBPW at Ropar are (i) the red ware; and (ii) they grey ware. Of the two, the red ware forms the dominant industry. Broadly, it is divisible into two categories slipped and unclipped red ware. The slipped red ware are generally of fine fabric; on some sherds, the slip een appear bright red. The unslipped red ware is largely from medium to coarse fabric, sometimes with gritty core. There is no exclusive shape confined to one category of the ware. Concerning pottery tradition, it will be relevant to mention here that there are some pottery shapes of the preceding period, i.e., Period II of the Painted Grey Ware culture, which continue into the Period III without any observable break in their tradition. These types from Period II are illustrated in the context of Period III., and not again from Period III to avoid repetion (Fig. 2).

The main red ware shapes in the period under discussion are bowls, basins with the without lug or loop handless, vases, pear-shaped jars, carinated *handis,* beakers, *Kulhar* like pots, miniature vessels and lids of different shapes and sizes (Figs. 3 and 4). Among them there are many shapes which alongwith their variants, occur at Hastinapur, Ahichahatra, Kausambi, Prakash, Vaisali, Taxila, etc. In additional to these, there are some new interesting types at Ropar like pottery mortar, *Kulhar* like vessels, etc., which are not reported from other sites.

Compared to red ware, the occurance of associated grey ware at Ropar is relatively less, with only limited shapes, but almost throughout the period. The grey ware is both of fine and coarse variety with or without slip. The sherds of fine fabric have thin section. However, no grey ware sherd has shown any painting or any kind of decorative design on them. The thick grey ware sherds, in some cases bearing dark-grey slip, are supposed by Sharma to be representing the devolution of the Painted Grey Ware sherds.

The main shapes in the Grey Ware, which are essentially utilitarian, are small and lare bowls, rim less *handi-s,* spouted jar, lids with central knob etc. Some similar shapes among these are also known to have reported from Hastinapur and Ahichchhatra.

As expected save for one (or two?) black and red ware sherds, which are opined by some as the accidental product of pottery firing, no cultural representation of black and red ware has been found at Ropar. Similarly, leaving a few grey ware sherds bearing black slip, no evidence of black slipped ware as such has been recorded from the excavations at Ropar.

Archaeological Survey of India,
Janpath, New Delhi.

K.C. NAURIYAL

REFERENCES

Indian Archaeology 1954-55 *A Review*

Lal, B.B. 1954-55. in *Ancient India*. 10 & 11: 4-151.

Panigrahi, K.C. 1946. in *Ancient India*. 1: 40-55.

Sahaya, S. 1969. Origin and Spread of the Northern Black Polished Ware. In *Potteries in Ancient India*. B.P. Sinha (ed.): 145-154.

Sharma, G.R. 1960. *Excavations at Kausambi. 1957-59*. Allahabad.

Sharma, G.R. 1969. *Excavations at Kausambi. 1949-50.* memoir 74. ASI.

Sharma, Y.D. 1956. Past Pattern in living as unfolded by excavations at Ropar. *Lalit Kala.* 1-2 New Delhi: 9-21.

Sinha, B.P. & S.R. Roy. 1969. *Vaishali Excavations.* 1958-62. Patna.

Sinha. K.K. 1969. The NBP Ware-Fresh Hypothesis in the light of Sravasti evidence. In *Potteries in Ancient India.* B.P. Sinha (ed.): 174-184.

Rock-Engravings at Tabo, Distt. Lahul and Spiti, Himachal Pradesh

Located within the Western Himalayan mountain system, village Tabo (Spiti) is well known for the largest monastery in Spiti valley, datable to circa tenth-eleventh century A.D. It is considered to be one of the most important centres of Buddhist learning, next only to Tholing Gompha in Tibet. In a recent exploration, rock engravings have been reported from this region. Tabo is situated about 50 kms south-east of Kaza, the Headquarters of District Lahul and Spiti, on the left bank of the river Spiti, a tributary of Sutlej. Located at an altitude of 3050 m and flanked on either sides by high mountains, it may be approached from Manali via Rohtang Pass, Kunzam Pass and Kaza and also from Shimla through Rampur Busher, Pipli and Sumdo. The route via Rohtang Pass, remains closed during winter because of heavy snowfall but Tabo remains approachable, throughout the year, from Shimla side, but for shot spells when the road is blocked by landslides and stone avalanches. Traditionally, Spiti was entered through, yet another route from Manali crossing the Hamta and Kunzam passes besides the ones which are being used even today. At Tabo the river has not changed its course since long as indicated by almost steep, northern river bank with absolutely no trace of any terrace. The river, presently flows about 30 m. below the flat surface of conglomerate deposit.

While exploring the area, close to the 108 stupa site (raised in a row), i.e., about 500 m east of the village, engravings on about forty boulders could be noticed (Pl. XXXII). These boulders, lying scattered on the flat ground, were fallen from the adjacent hill towards the north. Distributed in an area of about 1 sq. km., the boulders chosen for the engravings are not much larger in sizes and are embedded into the ground at varied depths.

Three groups of engravings have been observed on stylistic ground. The first group have been executed deep into the rock and exhibit extreme naturalism especially in case of animal depiction. the human forms, on the contrary, are abstract and reduced to schematic representations. These engravings have been executed with the help of sharp pointed tools. The execution of lines is fine in contrast to later engravings which are often drawn in wavering lines of varying thickness. It is rather difficult to understand the motivation behind repetitive representation of hunting scene. On majority of the boulders, the men have been depicted hunting the ibexes (wild goat) and sheep either by a solitary man or a group of two or more men. The heads of the hunters are club-shaped and the hands and the legs out-stretched in form of simple oblique lines. Even the body of the human forms has been indicated by drawing a vertical line below the head. the ibex has a pair of horns-curved backwards, four legs and again a curved tail (Pl. XXXIII). In some cases, the male genital organ, too, has prominently been depicted. The other animals shown through the engraving of this group, are the sheeps and dogs. The sheep may be easily identified from their bulky body and short legs. The dogs are small in size. The men engaged in hunting have, in majority of the examples, been portrayed holding bow and arrow or thirsting a long stick like weapon, almost similar to spear, towards the animal. The animals have, generally, been depicted in herds. The objects which are meant to be farthest have been shown smaller while those closer to the central figure are larger in size. The treatment of perspective has been given to the limbs of the standing animals which have been shown with four legs instead of two as the other two remain partly obscured by the ones closer to the viewer. This way of depicting the limbs has made the picture almost flat, particularly in those cases, wherein, the animal is shown not in motion Whenever, the animals have been shown in motion, it has given an added dynamism to the scene and the artist has been successful in expressing his feelings. But, these engravings suffer from a basic shortcoming of not being carved with any definite system as the artist has hardly taken any care to draw them following a pattern as various components of the scene fail to convey the relation between them. A careful examination of the engravings has revealed that all the pictures drawn on the surface of a boulder, were not only been executed by different artists but at different occasions also with considerable time-gap between them. One of the boulders is engraved with a group of three ibexes, a reindeer like animal with straight horns and an archer below, holding a bow in his left hand and an arrow in the right. The hunter has been shown readying himself to shoot an ibex, standing closeby. In an another scene, one can observe a man with a bow and arrow chasing a group of ibexes. At the bottom, two dogs have also been portrayed.

The depiction of woman, however, could be noticed in one example. She has a peculiar type of head, formed of two circles joined horizontally. The body is shown by drawing two vertical lines. Her hands projecting from the body towards her left have been shown holding a large unidentified object. The men and dogs, the other figurative depiction on the boulder, have been shown engaged in hunting the ibexes. Ponies also find depiction in one case alongwith earlier engravings of ibexes and men with bow and arrow, shown as hunters.

The engravings of the second group, classified purely on stylistic grounds, are those, wherein the animals have been portrayed in X-ray style, almost similar to the rock paintings. While the body of the animals have been drawn by double lines, the limbs continued to be represented through vertical lines. The horns, in case of ibexes, are shown curved on either sides of the head. However, the style of depicting other features of the animals is not much different from those of the first group. The subject matter also is almost the same as the men have been shown hunting the ibexes, except in one example. However, it is significant to point out that the style of portraying men has undergone a little change. The men have been shown sometimes with triangular head and body, and hands and legs outstretched. In other examples the human forms are represented in the manner similar to what has been employed in the group already discussed above. The men have, generally, been depicted hunting ibexes with bow and arrow. The representation of women appears to have deliberately been avoided suggesting their non-involvement in the hunting. One of the rock boulders is engraved with an animal which is unique as far as its representation is concerned. It has an open mouth, a pair of curved horns, tail curved upwards and two legs instead of four, one on the front and the other on the back. The engravings of this group appear to have been executed later than the first as indicated by the super-imposition, clearly visible on one of the boulders.

The engravings which are crude in execution and are not deep into the rock, have been classified into the third group. While the engravings of the earlier two groups centered around mainly hunting, those included in this group also portray groups of men standing in a row, snake biting a man, men and women in dancing posture, dogs and snakes. Occasional depiction of radiating sun, dots arranged in horizontal rows, trees and some unidentified symbols could also be noticed on the boulder surfaces.

One of the boulders depict a group of human forms most likely performing dance, as could be seen from the posture of their limbs. The scene depicted on entire rock surface comprises only two or three ibex figures. While the men have been represented in very simple forms, the women have been given a bit elaborate treatment as they have been shown with triangular heads. It is interesting to point out that the boulder bears a number of short inscriptions, engraved at the places which are free from pictorial depiction. The inscriptions in Brahmi characters, datable to circa fifth-sixth century AD seem to have been engraved earlier than the dancing scene as at one places the figures superimpose parts of the inscriptions. In an another example, a group of five men have been shown standing in a row. Towards their right, has been depicted, a screen sort of fence, and below, almost in its center, an ibex. It appears, the men are ambushing the ibex. The ibex shown on top, a sheep on the right and the radiating sun in the center, seem to have been engraved at a later date. The depiction of hunting scene, on an another boulder, is interesting as the human forms show variation in their style of execution. The men on left have outstretched horizontal hands and legs with vertical bends, from the elbow and knee joints, respectively, and a tail like appendage between the legs. The men, on the right and below, have club-shaped head, horizontally outstretched hands and legs. The hands have been shown bent at right angle from the elbow. Similar to the human forms depicted on the left, the men also have tails depicted on the left, the men also have tails depicted between the legs. dogs and sheeps are the other components of the scene. Crudely drawn ibexes are shown in the center in standing posture. Among the engravings of this group, a man holding a bow in his left hand and an arrow in the right raised upward above the head and the left leg forward shooting an ibex is one of the superb creations of the artist. A mythical snake with a pair of moustaches on the head, isolated depiction of tree, Svastika, ibexes, sheeps and dogs, of course rare, could be noticed. The artists were also aware to depict animals especially, the ibexes with completely filled body.

Apart from above some of the boulders bear depiction of human and animal figures in highly stylized forms. In some cases, these are superimposed over earlier engravings, indicating their execution at a later date. Simple and stylized depiction of *svastika* and a few indeterminate symbols could also be observed on a few boulders. One of such indeterminate symbols, enclosed within a circle, is associated with a four letter inscription in Brahmi characters. The inscriptions in Tibetan characters are also by no means rare.

In one example three stupas arranged almost on one horizontal plane have been found engraved. All the three rest over receding terraces, topped by chhatravali. The boulder is also engraved with a number of short inscriptions in Brahmi characters(Pl. XXXIV). Interestingly, traces of earlier engravings, depicting ibexes all over, could also be noticed on the boulder surface however, Buddhist deities are also engraved on some of the boulders (Pl. XXXV).

As far as the dating of these engravings is concerned is too premature to state anything conclusive due to lack of sufficient data. We can only suggest that those were executed at different periods. However, those depicting hunting scenes appear to be earlier in date than the ones bearing label inscriptions in Brahmi characters of *circa* fifth-sixth century A.D. The stupas were executed much later, sometimes around circa eleventh-twelfth century A.D.

It may not be out of place to mention that almost similar types of rock-engravings have been reported by A.H. Dani (1983) from Chilas, and Hunza located on the upper course of river on Karakoram Highway dated from circa fifth millennium B.C. to late medieval times. An extensive survey of the District along rivers Satluj (Distt. Kinnaur, H.P.), Spiti and Chandrabhaga (Distt. Lahul and Spiti, H.P.) may reveal similar rock engravings.

Archaeological Survey of India,
Janpath, New Delhi-110011.

A.K. SINHA

REFERENCES

Dani, A.H. 1983. Chilas: The city of Nanga Parvat (Dyamar). Islamabad

Report on the Chemical Analyses of the Glasses from Khairadih

Khairadih is situated in Ballia district of Uttar Pradesh on the right bank of river Ghaghara. Archaeological excavations were carried out during five sessions between 1981 and 1986 by the archaeologists of Banaras Hindu University. The excavations brought to light that existence of three successive cultural periods dated between c. 1100BC to AD300. The inhabitants of Period I (c. 1100 - 700BC) used black and Red ware, Black slipped ware, besides black burnished ware. Among important findings mention may be made of pendants and beads of carnelian, agate, chalcedony, blue-glass and disc shaped beads of steatite, terra-cotta beas and animal figurines. The use of copper is also attested. The Period II (700-200BC) is characterized by the occurrence of NBP ware, usage of iron, a glassmaking workshop - as evidenced by glass canes, unfinished beads and tiles, and copper coins. Apart from mud wall, burnt bricks were also used for making houses. Their Period III (200BC-300AD) is characterized by a spurt in building activities with significance of roads, drains and granary. The other findings consist of typical Kaushana coins, Kushana and Gupta style seals and sealings, beads of semi-precious stones, terra-cotta wheels and toy carts, utilitarian pots of iron and copper, unique pieces of red glass tiles and a great number of glass beads and bangles. (Singh 1989).

Materials and Methods

The objective of this study was to determine what chemical compositions or peculiarities might characterise the glasses excavated at Khairadih. From among the hundreds of specimens excavated, fifteen were selected for analyses. The sampling was not intended to be representative of the entire body of glass recovered. Instead, there was a strong bias in the sampling towards variety of glasses in colours and periods. A pieces of tile of copper-red colour was also selected for analyses which evidently represents fine quality of production. The sampling contains, apart from specimens of beads and bangles, a piece of gold-foil bead. This was the first analysis of any gold-foil bead in India. A piece of turquoise bead of central Asian origin was also subjected to the analysis for comparison with some of the glass beads.

The samples submitted for analysis were in most cases of a limited weight. For very small samples spectroscopic analysis was used, which gave approximate results for some chemical contents and required only a small quantity of powdered samples. Weights of the samples and the results of the analysis are given in the Tables I, II and III.

Results and Discussion

The data given in the Table II signifies that out of 15 samples of glass submitted for analysis only four i.e. KDH 280, KDH 1146/1, KDH 1767 and KDH 2262 had enough weight (more than 1.2 gm) which allowed to make a complete quantitative chemical analysis. The weight of the rest of the samples was enough only for spectroscopic analysis. On the basis of analysis one can establish approximately the glassforming components and in this way to categorise them according to the chemical types.

To the number of main glass forming components, we attributed those chemical oxides, the percentage of which in glass is three and more. Oxides which were added to the glass such as colouring agents and modifiers are not included in the number of glassforming components and are considered separately. If we use these parameters, we may attribute the samples from Khairadih to the following chemical types:

1. Na_2O-Al_2O_3-Fe_2O_3-SiO_2 Samples1, 2 (Table I)
2. CaO-Al_2O_3-Fe_2O_3-SiO_2 Samples 3 (")
3. Na_2O-K_2O-CaO-Al_2O_3-Fe_2O_3-SiO_2 Samples 4 (")

Thus, two types of glass belong to the first chemical type, consisting mainly of the oxides of sodium, alumina, oxide of iron and silica. The sum of these components in glass composition are 96.11 and 95.88 percent respectively. It is not possible at this stage to speak about full analogy of their compositions. Sample 1 is coloured by cuprous oxide and sample 2 by cupric oxide.

Another peculiarity of the first sample (No. 1) lies in the fact that copper are introduced into the composition of glass not as pure copper but as protoxide of copper. Composition signifies the presence of lead, iron arsenic, traces of nickel and cobalt (Table III) in a considerable quanitity.

The second sample (No. 2) consists of two parts KDH 1146/1 and KDH 1146/2. As it is seen from the Table I, both parts of the sample are considerably different in their chemical composition. The first part (1146/1) belongs to the glasss of type - Na_2O-Al_2O_3-Fe_2O_3-SiO_2, while the second (1146/2) to - Na_2O-CaO-MgO-Al_2O_3-Fe_2O_3-SiO_2. Samples 1 and 2, inspite of their resemblance to other glasses in chemical compositions and chemical types (except the occurrence of copper), are somewhat peculiar. They are distinct due to the higher percentage of alumina (18.90) and 17.49) and oxides of iron (11.70 and 14.74) in their composition. At the same time

Table I

Results of Chemical Analysis

Description	KDH 2880, piece of tile, copper red, opaque	KDH 1146, tiney bead, opaque black	KDH 1767, pieces of bangles, sky blue	KDH 2262 pieces of glass green sky-blue
Date	3rd Century B.C.	7th-2nd Cent. B.C.	7th-2nd Cent B.C.	1st-3rd Cent A.D.
SiO_2	60.85	59.40	70.17	69.85
Al_2O_3	18.90.	17.46	7.66	8.40
Fe_2O_3	11.70	14.74	3.43	3.29
TiO_2	0.10	0.10	0.09	NO
CaO	1.24	1.14	4.52	5.78
MgO	0.71	0.82	0.21	1.23
SO_3	NO	NO	NO	NO
MnO	traces	traces	0.01	0.01
K_2O	-	1.02	-	3.09
Na_2O	4.66	4.25	1.80	5.12
LOI	0.13	0.75	10.17	2.91
CuO*	-	0.29	1.95	0.35
Cu_2O	1.58	-	-	-

* Determined by difference, LOI = Loss on Ignition.

these two samples of glasses are characterized by a lower percentage of oxides of calcium (1.24 and 1.14) and oxides of sodium (4.66 and 4.25 respectively.

Obviously these samples were manufactured locally, because their compositions are more typical for Indian territory. Glasses with similar compositions are found from Arikamedu (2nd cent BC), Kopia (2nd cent BC), Kausambi (2nd cent. BC to 2nd cent . AD) and in some other places (Lal 1987; Brill 1987; Singh 1989). Lower percentage of alkali may be due to the leaching of glass during long burial under earth.

Table II

Description of Samples for Spectroscopic Analysis

Sample	Arch. No. KDH	Object	Colour	Date	Weight in gm
1.	1146/1	Tiny beads	Opaque with yellowish tint	VII-II-I Cent. B.C.	1.8
2.	1146/2	Pieces with shining surface	Blackish-opaque	"	0.6
3.	1569/1	Pieces of beads	Greenish	"	0.12
4.	1569/2	Pieces of glass	Grey-opaque	"	0.06
5.	1206	Pieces of bangles	Light-blue-opaque	"	0.47
6.	1767	"	"	"	1.50
7.	-	Piece of turquoise	Sky-blue	-	-
8.	2880	A small piece of tile of tile	Copper-red opaque	III Cent. B.C.	1.77
9.	278	A piece of bead bead (ring)	Greenish opaque	I-III Cent A.D.	0.13
10.	1094/1	A piece of gold-foil bead	Colourless with pinkish shade	"	0.20
11.	1094/1	A piece of glass with golden covering	"	"	0.20
12	1103	A piece of glass	"	"	0.12
13.	1767	A piece of loop or bangle	Colourless opaque	"	0.26
14	2262	A piece of glass	Greenish with blueish hue	"	1.21
15	2625/1	A piece of flat ring	Light blue	"	0.14
16.	2625/2	"	Greenish	"	0.18

Table III

Chemical Types of the Glasses

Sample No.	Chemical type of the glasses	Colourants and other components present > 1%
1.	$Na_2O-Al_2O_3-Fe_2O_3-SiO_2$	CuO
2.	$Na_2O-CaO-MgO-Al_2O_3-Fe_2O_3-SiO_2$	CuO
3.	$Na_2O-K_2O-CaO-Al_2O_3-Fe_2O_3-SiO_2$	-
4.	$Na_2O-K_2O-CaO-MgO-Al_2O_3-Fe_2O_3-SiO_2$	-
5.	$CaO-Al_2O_3-Fe_2O_3-SiO_2$	CuO
6.	$CaO-Al_2O_3-Fe_2O_3-SiO_2$	CuO
7.	$CaO-Al_2O_3-Fe_2O_3-SiO_2$	CuO
8.	$Na_2O-Al_2O_3-Fe_2O_3-SiO_2$	Cu_2O
9.	$Na_2O-CaO-Al_2O_3-SiO_2$	Cr_2O_3, PbO, P
10.	$Na_2O-K_2O-CaO-MgO-Al_2O_3-SiO_2$	(Au)
11.	$Na_2O-K_2O-CaO-MgO-Al_2O_3-SiO_2$	(Au)
12.	$Na_2O-K_2O-CaO-MgO-Al_2O_3-SiO_2$	Sb_2O_3 (Au)
13.	$Na_2O-K_2O-CaO-MgO-Al_2O_3-Fe_2O_3-SiO_2$	PbO, SnO_2
14.	$Na_2O-K_2O-CaO-Al_2O_3-Fe_2O_3-PbO-SiO_2$	PbO, SnO_2
15.	$Na_2O-K_2O-CaO-MgO-Al_2O_3-Fe_2O_3-PbO-SiO_2$	CuO, PbO, CuO
16.	$Na_2O-K_2O-CaO-MgO-Al_2O_3-Fe_2O_3-SiO_2$	CuO

The sample No. 3 (KDH 1767) stands quite distinct from all the glasses examined. This glass has nearly all glassforming oxides except the alkalies. Oxide of potassium is absent while the presence of sodium is very low, extremely high are the Loss of Ignition (LOI-10.17%). All these features make one doubt regarding the nature of the material. The glass was strongly weathered from which alkalies were depleted and their places were refilled by water, organic matters and soil solutions or it is a material of different origin, probably not a glass. As a rule such combination of chemical components are met among the ornaments made of turquoise. For comparison Table III (No. 8) gives spectral analysis of sky-blue turquoise from the central Asian region (Singh & Abdurajakov 1989). As it is close to the composition of sample No. 3 (KDH 1767).

Among the glass analyzed a special attention should be paid to the sample No. 4 (KDH 2262) in the Table I. According to the composition of the main glassforming components this glass belongs to the chemical type - $Na_2O-K_2O-CaO-Al_2O_3-Fe_2O_3-SiO_2$. Glass of this type but with a different combination of the main oxides were found in some of the early glasses in ancient India - Udaigiri (ancient period), Arikamedu, Kausambi and from other places (Singh 1989). But glasses with similar compositions with lower quanitity of oxides of iron were produced on a larger scale in Bactria especially during Kushana period. Recent studies have established the occurrence of such compositions in central Asia from N. Bactria, Old Termej, Dalverzintape, Surkhandarya, Surkh-Kotal, Kona-Maszid, Ak-Kupruk and in Afghanistan (Abdurajakov 1987). Thus, the distribution of this Kushana composition is established in Khairadih also.

In the last three samples (Nos. 2, 3, 4) the colours of glass and its hues are connected with the cupric oxide. The presence of small quantity of cobalt (i.e. 0.01% by spectral analysis) could not play any significant role in colouring.

The results from spectroscopic analyses are given in Table III. As it may be observed in most cases they prove the results of the chemical analysis and signifies the characteristics of glass under investigation to the previously established chemical types. On the basis of the results of spectral analysis of Khairadih glasses posses several new types (Table III).

Conclusion

On the basis of study of chemical compositions of 15 samples of glasses from Khairadih, it was established that they belong to 10 chemical types. Some were widespread in Indian contexts while others were found in central Asia and the Old-World. Naturally, it signifies the existence of ties between these centres and India in hoary antiquity.

On the other hand, the presence of a wide range of chemical compositions in glasses recovered from a single place and absence of any direct evidence of any connection with the Old-World, indicate the existence of indigenous and highly developed glass making centre at Khairadih, where the ancient people achieved remarkable advancement in glass manufacturing.*

Deptt. of A.I.H.C. and Arch.,
B.H.U., Varanasi.
Institute of Archaeology,
Uzbek Academy of Sciences,
Samarkand-57, U.S.S.R.

RAVINDRA N. SINGH AND
A.A. ABDURAJAKOV

REFERENCES

Abdurajakov, A.A. 1987. *Archaeometry of Glass* (H.C. Bhardwaj, Ed.). Calcutta: 40-41.

Brill, R.H. 1987. *Archaeometry of Glass* (H.C. Bhardwaj, Ed.) Calcutta: 44-56.

Lal, B.B. 1987. In *Archaeology of Glass* (H.C. Bhardwaj, Ed.). Calcutta: 44-56.

Singh, R.N. 1989. In *Ancient Indian Glass: Archaeology And Technology*. Delhi: 55-99.

Singh, R.N. and A.A. Abdurajakov, 1988. *Social Sciences in Uzbekistan. 8:* 66-72 (In Russian).

Singh, B.P. 1989. *Puratattva*. 18. 1987-88: 28-34.

Analytical Investigation of Indian Bronzes

Out of all the metals used by our ancestors, the most thoroughly investigated is copper and its alloys. Most of the works done on copper and its alloys relate to coins and analytical works on Indian bronzes is very scanty. Probably the holders of samples do not want to part with a few milligrams of samples required for analysis, but with the advent of non-destructive and rapid methods of analysis, this aspect has also been taken up. Due to recent restoration of theft sculptures of Tamil Nadu, it has become imperative to know the chemical composition of all our bronzes, so that the same could be confirmed. Analytical data will not only help in the identification of objects in case of theft or distinguish the object from the modern fake ones but will also give information on ancient metallurgy, provenance of ores etc., a problem most sought by archaeologists. An attempt has been made in this paper to collect information about the amount of work done on ancient Indian bronzes and the state of technology prevailing at that period of time. At the end, the analytical data obtained from the analysis of Angkor wat bronzes have also been included.

The first metals known to man were those occurring in the native state i.e. gold, copper and meteoritic iron. Discovery of other metals came at later dates. Beads of native copper from Tepe Ali Kosh (6500 B.C.) are the earliest known copper artifacts (Hole and Heizere 1969: 195). In the Indian sub continent copper metallurgy started during the Harappan period which slowed down during the central Indian Chalcolithic period and again picked up during Copper Hoard cultures. In the beginning unalloyed copper was the most popular metal but later on our ancestors learnt the importance of alloying the copper with other metals.

In the very early stage, metals mostly used for alloying copper were lead and tin. The bronze sculptures of 9-15th century have been found mostly alloyed with tin and lead. With the advent of zinc for the very first time from India, the pattern of alloying changed and most sculptures from 18 - 20th

* This paper has been partially presented in the international symposium on Archaeology, held at Heidelberg, Germany in April, 1990 by the first author.

century have been found alloyed with zinc along with lead and tin. But the amount of zinc used to alloy copper varies from place to place. Analysis report of Wearer shows that while more zinc was added to the copper in sculptures of Western India/ Northern India including Tibet, the amount of zinc added to sculptures of Southern India is either nil or very little. Zinc ore was first discovered from Jewar mines of Rajasthan and Western countries came to know about the metal zinc in later periods.

Long before tin was known, bronzes were in common use. In Egypt, Mesopotamia and Indus Valley, alloys of copper and tin were being produced in 3000 B.C. Tin is obtained from its ore cassiterite. Most of the tin from antiquity has perished either due to allotropic modification or has been oxidised to a mixture of stannous and stannic oxide. The only beneficial effect seems to have been used by our ancestrals due to alloying tin with copper was the increase in fluidity, workability and lowering of melting point. Pure copper melts at 1085°C whereas copper with 8%, 13%, 25% of tin melts at 1020°C, 980°C and 800°C respectively.

Different Groups

Indian bronzes can be divided into following groups depending on the addition of various metals/ non-metals to the copper

i) Bronzes with varying tin content ranging from 2 - 26%. In few bronzes upto 32% tin has been found.

ii) Copper-lead-tin bronzes in which in addition to copper and tin, lead has been added upto about 15%.

iii) Bronzes containing Arsenic, in Indian bronzes upto about 3%.

iv) Bronzes containing along with copper, tin and lead, a high amount of zinc (upto 20%) especially in later periods of 18 - 20th century.

Along with the above metals, ancient Indian bronzes are associated with a number of other elements which may be regarded as impurity from the ore or sometimes deliberate addition. The impurity varies with the type of ores used for smelting, the metallurgical process of extraction of the metals and refining process used.

The amount of iron is very high in most of the Indian bronzes and iron upto a concentration range of 0.13 to 2.57% have been reported. But on the other hand there are bronze objects with very low concentration of iron (0.01%-0.05%) which can be explained on the basis of difference in the types of ores used in smelting.

Nickel in most of the Indian bronzes are present in the concentration range of 0.01% to 0.66% except in few cases where nickel has been deliberately added. Sulphur is found in most of Indian bronzes which gives indication of the use of Sulphide ore of copper by our ancesters.

The other important elements found in Indian bronzes are arsenic and antimony. During roasting of ore most of the AS & Sb volatilize as As_2O_3 and Sb_2O_3 but some of these are converted to AS_2O_5 and Sb_2O_5 which are less volatile and form non-volatile arsenate and antimoniate with copper and hence amount of AS & Sb depends on the nature of atmosphere during roasting (Newton and Curtis 1942: 70). There are bronzes with concentration of arsenic upto about (0.1% - 1%) bronzes with concentration of arsenic upto about (0.1% - 1%) and antimony between (0.01 - 0.5%). In some bronzes arsenic has been added deliberately upto a concentration of 3%, copper arsenic alloys, though inferior to copper-tin alloys, are superior to pure copper in many ways, they melt more easily, are harder and produce sounder castings. The only way to obtain a high arsenic concentration would be either selecting copper minerals particularly rich in arsenic or by adding arsenic minerals to the smelting mix so as to get a copper of particular properties. But gradual discontinuation of the use of arsenic may be due to high toxicity of arsenic. Since copper-arsenical ores are not common occurrence in old world, it is interesting to find out the raw materials for rich arsenical bronzes. Silica in traces has been reported from Indian bronzes which may be regarded as impurity from the ore, sometimes silver has been added to bronze to give it an intrinsic value.

Results & Discussion

Bhardwaj has analysed some copper objects and copper slags belonging to 600 - 200B.C. and reported CaO and MgO in it which gives indication that probably lime and magnesia were used as flux in smelting process (Bhardwaj et al. 1968-69: 30-34). Some evidences of primitive smelting practices from Sikkim and Singhana near Khetri have been reported (Bose et. al. 1971: 300-301). Analysis of copper slag from Ahar has been reported by Agrawal quoting the views of K.T.M. Hegde's analysis of slag and indicates that silica might have been added as a flux (Agrawal 1971: 158). The presence of slag particles in the metal objects indicates that very clean separation of the slag and molten metal did not take place probably due to non-attainment of such a high temperature required for complete separation. Large number of studies on birth of copper metallurgy in India have been done by Agrawal. Kausambi bronze fragments (535-465B.C.) have been analysed and found to contain 79.12% Cu, 19.13% of Sn. Taxila copper (400 B.C.) has been found to contain 87.24% of Cu and 8.28% of Sn. Copper objects from Harappa have been analysed by Sanaullah and have been reported to contain about 10.45% of tin. Vats 1940: 378. C.H. Desch and E.S. Carvey have analysed samples of copper objects from Mohanjodaro and reported tin upto 26.9%. (Mackay: 1938: 480). V.. Smith ahs analysed bronzes of copper hoards and found it to contain 3.83% to 13.3% of tin (Smith 1985: 229). Wearer have analysed some copper objects from 16 - 18th century of Indian origin. He first found lead-tin-bronze with about 7% Sn. and 10% Pb. followed by lead tin-zinc alloy with about 4% Sn, 5% Pb and 5% zinc and lastly a similar alloy with about 2% Sn, 3% Pb and 17% Zn. This finding indicates about the addition of zinc only in later period. He also reported concentration of gold over 0.01% in Indian bronzes. Gradually the amount of gold decreases in the course of time and concentration below 0.005% occur in objects from 19th and 20th century. Lal, Paramasivan have also analysed copper objects and published reports in scientific journals.

V. Pandit Rao and P. Gayathri analysed some coins of Bahmani period and reported the addition of Sn & Pb in the early period of this dynasty which was discontinued from the middle of Bahmani period (Rao and Gayathri 1985: 27-44). Avadhanulu and Krishna Sastry showed that a definite ratio of Cu, Sn, Pb were present in copper coins of Sāatavāahana period (213 B.C. to 240 A.D.). A statuette of Lord Gaṇapathi has been analysed by Gayathri et. al. and found to contain Cu 660%, Sn 18%, Zn 15%, Fe. 2%, Pb 4% and Ni 0.8%.

Recently some bronze samples of Angkor Wat have been analyzed for its trace element contents first by emission spectrograph followed by Atomic Absorption spectrophotometer. The results obtained by me are given in tables 1 and 2.

TABLE - 1

Spectrographic analysis (in ppm)

Be Ga	Cu	Ag	Ni	Cr	Sn	Mo	Co	V	Nb	La	Y	Zn
<5 >5	in %	>1000	>1000	>10	in%	<300	<300	<10	<30	Cu	<10	<300
Sb As	Pb	Si										
<200	>1000	>1000	Traces							interference		

TABLE - 2

Atomic Absorption analysis of trace elements

Elements	Sample No. 1 12th Century	Sample No. 2 12th Century	Sample No. 3 11th cent.	Sam. No. 4 11th Century	Sam. No. 5 11th cent.	Sample No.6 16th cent.
Zn	40	60	34	288	24	244
Co	186	180	164	4	8	132
Ni	0.23 7%	0 .226%	952	324	270	688
Pb	0.2156 %	0.216	0 .30%	0 .71%	124	176
Bi	Nil	Nil	80	26	Nil	Nil
Sb	288	279	434	371	319	472
As	0.19 %	0.2 1%	880	0.18 %	0 .28%	462
Mo	108	40	Nil	Nil	20	Nil
Ag	0 .116%	0.11 6%	940	875	0.21 %	560
Si	Traces *	Traces *	Traces *	Traces *	Traces *	Traces *

* rest copper and tin

The difference in concentration of elements such as Ni, Pb, As, Ag from the samples of 11-12th Century to those of 16 - 19th Century is noteworthy.

From the above it seems that copper metallurgy in India did not pass from one culture to another completely.

M. SINGH

Archaeological Survey of India,
Hyderabad.

REFERENCES

Agrawal, D.P. 1971. The copper bronze age of India.
Bhardwaj, H.C. 1968-9. Rajghat - Copper a Metallurgical View. *Puratattva.* 2.
Bose, D.M. et. al. 1971. A concise History of Science in India.
Hole, F. and R.F Heizer. 1969. An introduction of Prehistoric Archaeology. New York.
Mackey E. 1938. Further Excavations at Mohenjodaro: 480.
Newton, J and L. Curtis. 1942. Metallurgy of Copper.
Pandit Rao, V. and P. Gayathri 1985. Journal of Arch. Chem. 3.
Smith, V.A. 1905. Indian Antiquary. 34.
Vats, M.S. 1940. Excavation at Harappa: 378.

World Archaeological Congress

Last year, the council of the World Archaeological Congress (WAC) accepted an invitation from its Indian members to hold its third congress (WAC 3) in New Delhi, late in 1994. The Government of India has recently given its approval and some financial support for this purpose, appointing the Archaeological Survey of India, the oldest and the most prestigeous archaeological organisation in South Asia, as the nodal agency for organising it.

Here, I should like to talk about some of the vital aspects of academic programme which will be considered by the Academic Planning Committee of WAC - India. They relate to the structure of the past World Archaeological Congress and have been the subject of preliminary discussions in U.K. between the WAC Secretariat and Professor V.N. Misra and Dr. Makkhan Lal, the delegates of WAC - India.

* * * *

Before I do this, however, I think it would be useful to say something about WAC and the new initiatives which it represents in the world of archaeology, not only in an academic sense, but as regards wider aspects of the discipline.

WAC is a young organisation, formally inaugurated in 1987, but dating its birth from 1986, when a Congress being organised in Southampton (UK) for the International Union of Pre- and Protohistoric Sciences (IUPPS) was disowned by the Executive Committee of that organisation because of the anti-aparthid stand taken by the British Organising Committee in banning South African participation. The Southampton Congress, even before it was disowned, had planned to be a meeting with themes and participation of a wide-ranging and international character, never achieved by its erstwhile parent body, either before or subsequently. The principles that were established at the Southampton Congress, now known as W.A.C.'s First Congress (WAC 1), from which more than 20 volumes of proceedings have already appeared, were continued at W.A.C.'s Second Congress (WAC 2) in Barquisemeto, Venejuela, in 1990 and are recommended for consideration in the organisation of the Third Congress (WAC 3) in New Delhi in 1994.

There are two basic concepts to be noted:

1. The first concerns the academic character of its meetings. Besides highlighting aspects of the archaeology of the host region, there are built around major themes in the disipline which will benefit from comparative discussion in an international perspective and to which archaeological experience from different parts of the world can contribute. Such themes in past WAC meetings have included patterns of domestication, pastoralism and predotion, problems in the study of tropical agriculture, the emergence and development of social hierarchy, the processes of innovation, the origins of human behaviour, and material culture and symbolic expression. It follows that if these universal themes are truly to draw on world experience in their investigation, participation by the world community of scholars is essential and WAC, as an organisation, sets itself the task of ensuring effective attendance by less advantaged countries.

2. W.A.C.'s second basic principle is that archaeology as a discipline has connectins, consequences and implications in the wider world in which it is situated. Indeed there is a vast range from matters like the management of the archaeological heritage in midern world, where it is under threat from things like increased economic development and illicit export of antiquities to the educational role of archaeology in the wider community and the appropriate presentation of its results in museums and school curriculoe. Underlying all is the important matter of the relationship of archaeology - and archaeologists - to the different cultural traditins on which its work impinges and the values of the communities amongst whom it is carried out. In these respects, WAC has sought to involve representatives from such traditions and communities in discussions of ethical guidelines for archaeological investigation, especially in the matter of skeletal remains about which aboriginal groups, particularly in North America and Australia have been much concerned. Agreed codes of conduct in these areas have been published in issues of the World Archaeological Bulletin (WAB).

* * * *

WAC welcomes the opportunity to hold its next Congress in India, because of the extreme richness of the Indian archaeological and cultural heritage and India's long experience for more than a century, in its large-scale investigation and highly organised management. We are conscious also of India's role in cooperative projects beyond her borders, including highly professional advice and assistance given in archaeological explorations and excavations in Nubia and Bahrain, and conservation of monuments in Afghanistan, Cambodia and other countries.

* * * *

The wider South Asian region of which India forms part, has a distinctive place in Old World history, as a link from the beginning between East and West. Following an initiative of our second Congress in Venezuela (WAC 2), we would encourage the Indian Academic Planning Committee to schedule for the opening day of the third Congress a series of presentations on the archaeology of South Asia for the benefit of the numerous foreign participants whom we expect the Congress to attract.

The following days of the Congress (four days of academic meetings and a day in the middle for local visits of archaeological interest) would see discussion broaden out into wider themes in which the regional experience will be important.

There may be some specialised post-congression sessions at places other than that of the congress. some of these will appropriately relate directly to the South Asian scene. Topics which have been suggested include recent Advances in South Asian Archaeology, the study of the Indus Valley Civilization and long distance Trodl, Archaeology of Ancient Indian Language and Traditions, Ideology and Archaeology Art and Architecture of ancient religious and cultural traditions, the study of epigraphy and numismatics and problems of dating.

Following precedent, these would take the form of symposia, with contributed papers. The Academic Planning Committee of WAC - India would be responsible for their organisation. It would be likely to modify and add to the list given above and no doubt would be willing to receive further suggestions.

As regards what we may call the international themes of the Congress, the following suggestions have been made at Southampton to the Academic Planning Committee of WAC - India for its consideration.

1. The Neogene: Human colonization of the World, its environmental contexts, chronological aspects and technological evolutions.
2. Change in Agrarian System, which might look at the circumstances - in the plant, in the environment or in the society - under which some plants become staples, other potential staples do not, and some plants are replaced as stables by others.
3. Archaeology as an Indicator of Trade and Contact, which would explore problems in the interpretation of exotic materials and traits in the archaeoogical record (as well as problems posed by the disappearance of evidence from that record).
4. Technological Innovation and Power: what are the implications of technical innovation as revealed by archaeology in different socio-economic contexts for the exercise of power - its acquisition, consolidation or loss.
5. State and Society, which would continue previous WAC discussions in exploring questions of the origin and development of social hierarchy and its political concomitants.
6. Changing perspectives in Historical Archaeology, which is a rapidly develoing branch of our discipline, where the archaeologicl approach is brough to bear on issues in more recent history, of which the archaeology of colonial settlement is one.
7. Landscape Archaeology, discussing theory and method in the study and interpretation of archaeologial landscapes.

8 Archaeological Theory and Practice, which would explore the extent to which the rapidly growing body of theory in archaeology is usefully related to what archaeologists actually do.

9. Lanaugage and Archaeology, a theme of world-wide interest and important, given added relevance by recent publications about the origin and spread of Indo-European languages and the peoples who spoke them in terms of their cultures and physical types and the discussions they have stimulated.

10. Ethno-archaeology, broad theme that continues to attract attention in efforts to achieve more 'faithful' understanding of pat societies and whose treatment would include considration of th responses of the living societies under study.

11. Concepts of Time, which would look at the implications of the dating revolution achieved by increasing powerful scientific techniques for our understanding of past, but also at cultural attitudes towards time in the traditions of different societies, together with the role of education in the two fields and between them.

12. Cultural Property, Public Awareness and conservation of heritage, theme whose importance and urgency needs no stressing and whose Congress treatment - together indeed with other themes where relevant - would integrate three basic concerns of WAC as an organisation: the use of modern information technologies; model codes of conduct; the role of education; and the need to consider and consult the interests of the various communities for whom the cultural property is a matter of permanent identity and inseparable ethos deeply rooted in history, tradition and mythology.

* * * *

This list will no doubt be refined during its consideration by the Academic Planning Committee of WAC-India and probably added to by it and as a result of suggestions made to it. Once ateme has been adopted, its specificaiton in detail and its organisation will be the responsibility of an Indian Convenor (or convenors) working with one or two overseas scholar appropriate for the task.

It is hoped that the first announcement of the Congress, specifying themes and symposia and the names of at least some of their organisers, will appear in the early months of 1992, to be widely distributed in India and abroad.

I commend the Congress to you and invite your participation.

JACK GOLSON

President,
World Archaeological Congress
Professor, Prehistory Research,
School of Pacific Studies,
Australian National University,
Canberra, Australia.

BOOK REVIEWS

M.L. Varadapande, *Mahābhārta in Performance*, Clarion Books, New Delhi 1990, PP. 128 with 56 illustrations, Price 345/-.

The Indian theatre comprising dance, drama and music consecrated to the wills of dancing deities (nṛtyamāno Devatā. Rg. 5-33-6) nucleated in the inspiration of the sages through divine damsels (apsarases) and gandharvas who met to perform plays in celestial groves or the Indra's Paradise.

Traditions of such inspirational instincts of entertainment and bliss in Indian history and fiction are known from the mesolithic rock engravings, murals, rituals and literary compositions beginning with the dialogue hymns in the Vedas and heroic stories of the *Rāmāyaṇa* and the *Mahābhārata* which while enlarging our vision of the rich culture heritage provide unmistakable evidence against the antiquity of the Greek drama to its Indian counterpart. The Greek drama doth go only to Europedes' satyr *Cyclops* or Aristophanes's presentation of his comedy *The Wasps* shown at the Lenaean festival of 422 B.C., an erotic kordax with lewd denudation; likewise Aeschylus (525-456) wrote the first European drama in 492 B.C. Similarity is met with in the modality of recitation by bards, the Indian sūtas and the Greek 'Choros' (celtic > bard, in Latin, bardo) alongwith some other features of the inevitable disposition and crisis of actors as their positive and negative energies coil up in turmoil.

The author presents a long standing tradition of Indian theatre in complete assurance of the arts, artists and audience in their theatrical and human *savoir-faire*. The themes discussed here are : 1. The Epic, 2. Early Performances, 3. Bhāsa, 4. Kālidāsa, 5. The Kṛṣhṇa Saga, 6. The Pāṇḍava Vāṇī, 7. Terukkuttu, 8. South Indian Dance Drama, 9. The Modern Era and 10. The Brook Experiment. The exhaustive bibliography at the end of the work gives information about the critical editions of the Mahābhārata in regional languages and as many as 56 suggestive illustrations instill art awareness.

In his studies of Bhāsa and Kālidāsa he has restructured the rhetorical techniques and far-spread impact of the *Mahābhārata* on visual arts.

The anecdotal image presented in the context relates to the seven plays of Bhāsa: 1. *Madhyama Vyāyoga*, 2. *Pañcarātra*, 3. *Dūta Vākya*, 4. *Dūtaghaṭotkaca*, 5. *Karṇābharaṇam*, 6. *Urubhaṅgam* and 7. *Bālacaritam*, which are glimpsed from the viewpoint of dramatic art.

Likewise, the two famous plays of Kālidasa *Vikramorvaśīyam* and *Abhijñāna Śakuntalā* based on the *Mahābhārata* have been critically examined to vouchsafe their romantic and poetic traditions particularly the latter which appearing for the first time on the German stage (1789) discombed the classical canons in Europe.

Foremost among Sanskrit poets both Bhāsa and Kālidāsa were great innovators who moderated their themes to produce the dramatic and literary effects. The tradition of Bhāsa's plays has continued in the service of the classic Kutiyattam plays of the chakyars of Kerala. Kālidāsa has put the cerebral concepts of the legends into very vital substance of reality in lyrical style.

Drama with dance, music, costumes and masks, often in the form of chorus and marionette has been quite popular in India, performed as the kaṭhaputalī (Rajasthan), Kathak (U.P.), Maṇipurī (Assam), Sakhi Kundhei and Odissi (Orissa), Gombeyata (Karnataka) imitating the Yakshagānam actors who play the episodes of the *Rāmāyaṇa* and *Mahābhārata*. In similar ways the epics are dramatised by Chhau dancers of Orissa and the naṭs, marionette actors of the Bastar region and the rāsa of Mathura, the Gujarati Garaba and Rathayātrā (car procession) during the Ratha-festival of Lord Jagannātha. Other regional plays are no exception.

The South Indian traditional dance dramas of Karanatak Kathakali Yakshagānam and Terrukkuttu present the most animated scenarios.

The Yakshagānam is essentially dominated by the *Mahābhārata* as its repertoire consists of such themes as Kṛṣṇārjuna-Kalag, Abhimanyu-Kalag, Draupadī Svayaṁvara, Bhīshma Parva, Rājasūya, Subhadrā Kalyāṇam with all the traits of the invocational style and elegance of Bhāratnāṭyam. These plays are based on *Harivaṁsa* and the *Bhāgavat* and as performed with orchestral music enthrall the audience.

Terukkuttu, an open air musical opera initially starting with the Tamil classic *śilappādhikāram* is associated with the Draupadī Amman festival. It is interesting that the Kaṭṭiakkaṛan (Sūtradhāra and jester as one) is always present on the stage participating in the drama.

The *Kṛṣṇa Saga* and *The Pāṇḍava Vāṇī* are two analogical categories of performing arts based on the Kṛṣṇa's lore and further *Mahābhārata* episodes. The author discusses the thematic basis of the texture and content of the Kṛṣṇa theatre and refers to various choreographic compositions.

The ballad singers of *Maharashtra* are known for recital of Pāṇḍava Vāṇī and belong to two classes, 1. the Kathakas and 2. the Kapilakas. Recitation of ballad is a common place thing in the entire sub-continent. The tribals of Assam and the jonsar-Bavar region have engrafted their own peculiarities in the recitations, while the *Mahābhārata* stories are narrated in the *Kathakalākṣepam* musical story events and the *Kathācakras* in Tanjavur.

Many näive interpretations of scholars as to origin of Indian theatre and criticism of drama who are unable to see through the intercession of divine powers in men's affairs galvanizing them into action by assuming human forms, creating such phantasmagoria as embryos moving from womb to womb, manifestation of incarnations and the other *elemento miracolo* have been skillfully answered by Varadpande.

Coming to our own time the author analyses the effects of *Mahābhārata* plays in the Marāṭhi theatre, particularly as the drama of 'Kīchaka-vadha' which witnessed by Lokamanya Tilaka, Aurobindo and Lajpat Rai created commotion in public (vide *Times of India*, Feb. 5, 1910).

But a more viable and universal appeal is sought in the Brook Experiment in the modern era. It is a theme of Peter Brook's theatrical production of the *Mahābhārata* scripted by Jean Claude Carriere and inspired by the traditional dance, drama of Karanataka *Kathakali Yakshagānam* from which it notably varies in technical art and demonstration. In its plainness and exquisite impressiveness it shadows the Hollywood scenarios depicting old fables or woesome movies as David Lean's *The Bridge on the River Kwai* or *Ryan's Daughter.* Jack Kroll saw a combination of Homeric Poems and Complete Shakespeare in Brook's opera.

The impact of the *Mahābhārata* has been indelible on men's minds throughout the world. Thus, 'right from Bhāsa and Kālidāsa to Bhaṭṭa Nārāyaṇa' says Varadpande,' and further to the composers of the Terukkutu plays everybody not only used the *Mahābhārata* and connected primary related secondary and extended myth material but creatively added to it or changed it to serve their dramatic ends. Sometimes, as we see, these changes are on a superficial level but many a time they are quite radical and all pervading even to the extent of creating altogether a new version of the *Mahābhārata*.

The Mahābhārata in its imaginatively diversified forms, from the dialogue format and narrative frame to bas reliefs and murals and all creative works including the performing arts has moved the world with its three immortal precepts, restraint, renunciation and rectitude which lead to bliss (MBH XII-V. 43-22).

Highland Cottage, C. MANI
Mussoorie.

Anatoly I. Martynov. *The Ancient Art of Northern Asia*, University of Illinois Press, Urbana and Chicago, 1991, pp. 300 including figures and plates 147, Price ....

In this comprehensive work, the author has discussed until now the poorly known Siberian archaeological art from the Paleolithic to medieval times. Basically the history of north Asia which is a zone of unwritten history, has been handled by the author by dividing it into six chapters, namely, the Paleolithic Neolothic, Eneolithic-Early Bronze, Scytho-Siberian and Medieval. The last chapter on the tree and life has integrated a good part of the preceding material.

The chapter one deals with the art of mammoth hunters. The Stone age is divided into two chronological periods - Lower and Middle Palaeolithic. In the upper Palaeolithic times there were several cultures with their own traditions of stone working. In this period the sites of Malta culture are quite distinctive. The female statuettes of varying shapes and bird sculptures from this place are different from analogous European figurines. The chapter on Sacred animals and Solar symbols represents the pursuit of mammals into the mesolithic, neolithic and early bronze ages. In fact, the Neolithic art was a continuation of the basic traditions of palaeolithic realistic art. However, the moose became the major image of north Asian art.

The chapter three on Three eyed idols and enigmatic masks deals with the north Asian art during the palaeometallic epoch i.e. eneolithic and bronze ages. The Bronze age which is represented by several genres, contributed a common ideology and religion among the ancient steppe tribes. The ideology embodied the cults of Sun, Sacred animals and the Nature. The next chapter on the Golden reindeer and flying to the Sun, deals with Steppe Culture and development of Scytho-Siberian art, whereas in Chapter five the consequence of the great migration of peoples in northern Asia during the second and first centuries B.C. has been discussed. The last Chapter traces the artistic handling through time of a major mythological theme, the Tree of Life.

In conclusion, the author has observed that the art of northern Asia did not emerge casually and independently of the broader history of mankind.

The work which has been translated and edited by Demitri B. Shimkin and Edith M. Shimkin deserves all praise for making this valuable data available to scholars using English.

Archaeological Survey of India,
Janpath, New Delhi. K.N. DIKSHIT

O. Guillaume Analysis of *Reasonings in Archaeology* Oxford University Press, Delhi, 1990, pp. 133, figures 33, tables 4, Price Rs. 128/-.

The book deals with Bactro-Indo-Greek (BIG) numismatics. Essentially, the author examines two main contributions - of Tarn The Greeks in Bactria and India and of Narain (The Indo-Greeks). It is, a bit enigmatic as to why the author did not include these works in his bibliography.

The author in all his sincerity tries to introduce some objectivity and scientific methodology in the study of numismatics and the interpretations derived. He points out that Tarn and Narain's conclusions on many points are not only different but sometime absolutely contradictory. This difference is not explained away just by the discovery of the new coins by the time Narain produced his study. The differences lie in the interpretation of identical sources. Tarn stressed the Greek contribution to BIG history and Narain, on the other hand, plays it down. The differences therefore are ideological. Guillaume uses the theoretical framework of Gardin's book, *Archaeological Constructs -An Aspect of theoretical Archaeology*. The author thus sets his present study in the framework of logicist analysis. Step by step, Guillaume lays down the scientific criteria underlying the study of numismatics. He defines the *Corpus,* he lists the variables for describing the coins, and lays down rules for classifying the coins. He then goes on to study the historical constructions based on numismatic data with reference to BIG history. He provides an inventory of reasonings based on a number of parameters about variations in material, overstrike, type and royal portraits and in legends.

The author concludes that both Tarn and Narain's works would fall in the category of narrative history. Guillaume finds that both Tarn and Narain use categorico-deductive approach rather than hypothetico-deductive. The author laments that the historian soon forgets that the premises on which he bases his reconstruction have hypothesis status and he tells them not to consider them as well established truth from which he deduces true conclusions. For example, overstrike could signify conquest or metal shortage. But the author chooses one and takes it as a proven truth and then bases the construction on such hypothesis. He therefore pleads that all hypotheses should be confronted with facts to verify them. The author concludes that any progress in BIG historiography is inevitably linked to the establishment of topology on the basis of the variables used by the catalogues in their descriptions of coins. It is a safe bet that a fair number of hypotheses put forward by the historians will then collapse. The author is not trying to be negative but provides a methodology to bring in scientific objectivity in the study of numismatics.

As far as the book is concerned, it brings in a fresh breeze and a new vigor into the discipline of numismatics. All laymen and scholars interested in the study of archaeology, coins, history and historiography benefit from it. It is good to see the profound contributions of French scholars now opening upto the English knowing readers.

Physical Research Laboratory D.P. AGRAWAL
Ahmedabad.

B.R. Mani. *The Kushan Civilization*, B.R. Publishing Corporation, Delhi, 1987, pp. 276, plates 36, Price Rs. 160/-.

In the present work, the author has analysed the data to explain material forces responsible for the development of socio-economic structure in the Kushan times. The study which is divided into six chapters is supported by appendices and a detailed bibliography. It traces the history of Kushans from the Central Asian steppes in Oxus zone to their new home in India. He has made an indepth study of the art and architecture of Kushans including the numismatology, organisation of government, industrial growth and external trade of the period. The chapters on society and culture, crafts and the economic activity have been dealt with in detail. The archaeological evidences have also been taken into account but they have their own limitations due to non publication of reports. The presence of a large building noticed at Sirsukh (Taxila), is an evidence of granary constructed in a Kushan town. The Kushans were also responsible to popularize a heavy diaper masonry as can be seen in different stupas and monasteries at Taxila and also in the buildings at Charsada. In Ganga valley, they used bricks frequently.

However, the author is right in his observation that in this period the wide cultural assimilation and unity which accelerated an alround development of civilisation in many fields has taken their firm roots. They were so much influenced by the Indian sentiments and cultural heritage that their process of assimilation though not sudden or radical became a reality. The Kushans also initiated the Scythic era of A.D. 78 which is still recognised in India as national era (śaka-saṁvat).

This book is an important contribution towards understanding the urban-development stages and material culture of Kushan civilisation.

Archaeological Survey of India, K.N. DIKSHIT
Janpath, New Delhi.

Gopal Narayan Bahura and Chandramani Singh. *Catalogue of Historical Documents in Kapad-Dwara*, Jaipur, Part II: Maps and Plans Jaipur, 1990, pp. 168, plates XXXVI, figures 67, Price Rs. 500/-

The book deals with old maps and plans in the collection of Pothikhana, City Palace Museum, Jaipur. As many as 372 rare maps and plans mostly prepared in the eighteenth century have been classified which illustrate parts of the world, Indian subcontinent showing many historical cities, places of pilgrimage viz. Jaipur, Jodhpur, Ajmer, Ujjain, Delhi, Puri, Dacca, Pushkar, Varanasi, Prayag etc. The contents reveal astronomical drawings, forts, geographical maps, gardens, dams, rivers, water canals, havelis, palaces, military campaigns, cannons, hunting scences and indoor games labelled with inscriptions in Devanagari and Arabic scripts. These inscriptions have been deciphered and a glossary of terms added for readers not conversant with Rajasthani dialects. Some of these maps were acquired or prepared at the instance of kings and chieftains of Jaipur state to acquaint themselves with various parts of country and territory, whereas some were used for settling boundary disputes.

During the rule of Maharaja Ram Singh of Amer (1667-1688 A.D.) Bihar, Orissa and Bengal (including areas of Bangla Desh) were surveyed and maps got prepared by devoted cartographers on large sized cloth. These maps in Kapad-Dwara collection are unique contribution to geographical history. While inspecting various forts and medieval cities of Rajashtan as an officer of the Archaeological Survey of India, I have experienced that many constructions or their parts which could not be precisely dated for want of direct evidence could now be securely dated, reassessed and associated with specific events with the help of these drawings as the stylistic analysis alone could not be the deciding factor. To cite an example of Ranthambhor fort, a monument of national importance, temple of Sita Ramji, Zanana Palace, twentytwo pillared chhatri, Rao Duda's Kuchery etc. owing to map No. 255 (not illustrated owing to fragile condition of the cloth texture) gives a clear idea of additions and alterations which took place in the fort after it came in the possession of Jaipur ruler Madho Singh in 1754 A.D. Another map shows that a brick wall around Surat city was constructed after 1666 A.D. because the previously built mud wall was seen by the European Traveller, Thevenot. This book would prove to be a useful tool for archaeologists and historians studying palaces, forts and town planning of medieval cities of Western India.

Archaeological Survey of India, P.K. TRIVEDI
Jaipur Circle, Jaipur.

V.R. Mani Sons of *Śiva A study in the Religious cults of Gaṇeśa and Kārttikeya*, Sharda Prakashan, Delhi 1990, pp. 96, Price Rs. 130/-.

The pioneering works on Hindu iconography by Gopinath Rao and J.N. Banerjee opened a new vista in the field of iconological studies. While collating the traditional sources with iconographical material, they impart an insight into future researches for a deity-wise study. With the passage of time such studies made advances with archaeological material right from the historical period to the late medieval times. In recent past several good research papers and monographs have appeared on the iconography of sons of Śiva. Basically these researches have touched upon the question of genesis, and analyse the process of iconographic development wherever possible with the help of available material and tradition.

The present monograph on the sons of Śiva falls short of iconographic details; It has, besides the introductory note, chapters on Gaṇeśa and Skanda-

Kārttikeya-Murugan. The introduction discusses Aiyappan considered to be the third son of śiva according to the late traditions of peninsular India.

The chapter on Gaṇeśa deals with issues like origin, Paurāṇic traditions, known archaeological facts, and finally the cult of Gaṇeśa in Tamil country getting more space for discussion than the one noted above. Similarly, the chapter on Kārttikeya, subdivided on the above lines, treats the iconographic aspects of Murugan in a lucid manner, while the discussion on Skanda-Kārttikeya remains too sketchy to perceive. On the contrary, the variety of illustrations used in the monograph provides a wide spectrum for discussion with regard to the process of development and regional variations and traditional myths attached to some of these forms.

AMARENDRA NATH

Archaeological Survey of India,
Excavation Branch, Nagpur.

Lallanji Gopal. *The Economic Life of Northern India c. A.D. 700-1200,* Motilal Banarsidass Publishers Private Limited, Delhi, 1989, 2nd Edition, Price Rs. 150/-. pp. 327.

The present work is the Ph.D. thesis of the author for which he received degree from the London University. It was completed under the guidance of A.L. Basham and was first published in 1965. The second edition which has been published without any change has two new appendices dealing with the "Samanta - tis varying significance in Ancient India" and the "Techniques of Agriculture". The first edition was well received by the students and scholars of economic history. It is good that, now, we have its second edition made available at a reasonable cost.

The new material in the form of appendices is very useful. The first note analyses the term *Sāmanta* as related to the genesis and change in the status of the sāmants alongwith the etymological significance of the term.

The presentation of the analysed data reflects clarity and erudition of the scholar. But at certain points the students would certainly like to seek his comments in more precise terms. For example, he quotes Vijñāheśvara, a commentator of 12th century A.D., as saying that '*Sāmanta* means the villagers living on the four sides. But then he also cites Somadeva's *Kathāsaritsāgara,* a text of 11th century A.D. in which the said term denotes a chieftain or noble having the right to enjoy some fixed income. Thus the reason for which Vijñāneśvara does not give the contextual meaning of the term, pertaining to his own period, should have been discussed in detail.

The other note (in Appendices) describes the agricultural techniques. It fulfils the requirement of the main thesis. A monograph on the economic life of Indian people without an account of agricultural process must certainly appear incomplete, particularly when the ownership of land is discussed in detail. The information contained in this appendix is, therefore, very important. It tells almost all the problems related to irrigation, the scientific consideration concerning the soil, manure, seed and sowing. It also discusses the nature of agricultural implements, etc., on the basis of the literary texts of various types and inscriptions. The enrichment of the bibliography with further readings and studies in the revised edition would have much added to the corelative significance in the area of economic research.

Jammu University, Jammu. Y.B. SINGH

Urmila Sant. *Neolithic Settlement Pattern of North-Eastern and Northern. India,* Sarita Book House, Delhi, 1991, pp. 41. Figures 19, Plates I-XLVI, Price Rs. 600/-.

It is a well documented work on the neolithic man in India although in the past A.H. Dani and T.C. Sharma produced authenticated monographs on this subject specially on north eastern India. The work has been thoughtfully designed into five chapters. The settlement pattern of Excavated Sites - Chapter IV which has been dealt state-wise has thrown valuable light on the neolithic evolution in India and its distribution pattern specially in eastern India. An attempt has also been made to co-relate neolithic artifacts with environment. However, the author's observaton that in the Gangetic Doab, the neolithic way for emergence of cities requires an analytical study of archaeological data as the developmental stage between the end of neolithic and the beginning of Iron Age has still to be worked out because the process of urbanisation in Ganga valley is far from clear.

However, in writing this kind of work the author must have faced many restraints as most of the work done in eastern India has remained unpublished. And so is the case with the principal neolithic excavated site in northern India. Due to this difficulty, the analytical cross section of neolithic settlement pattern of different regions could not be studied in detail and rather make it difficult to draw sound observations at many places.

This work with the help of plates and figures has provided extremely useful data.

Archaeological Survey of India, Janpath, New Delhi. **K.N. DIKSHIT**

Prakash Sinha, *Model for Land-use in Late Acheulian Tradition* (Satna District, M.P.), Prayag Pustak Sadan, Allahabad, 1991, pp. 224, with figures and plates,

This is indeed the first attempt in India to retrieve subsistence activities of the Late Acheulian man through a statistical model as the study of Lower Palaeolithic is relatively more complex than the later cultures. The book which is divided into seven chapters is supported by three appendices. The Chapter on Methodology and Terminology provides information about the nature of sites and attributes of artifacts and also explains the concept of statistical model, whereas the chapter on Analysis which has been classified under four heads has provided all the relevant material necessary for understanding the identification of probable relationship between the sites and regions. The last chapter deals with discussion and observations on some of the major problems raised and investigated in the present work.

While comparing the assemblage recovered in the study area, a three fold typo-technological stratification has been proposed for the Acheulian tradition in India. The author who has laid emphasis on sampling methods supported by tables and figures, has attempted to explain the rationale behind the variation in the dimension of sites and their location.

This work has contributed a new approach to the subject and would serve as a model for similar works.

Archaeological Survey of India, Janpath, New Delhi. **K.N. DIKSHIT**

INDIAN ARCHAEOLOGICAL SOCIETY

RECEIPTS AND PAYMENTS FOR THE YEAR ENDED 31.03.1991

ACCOUNTS

By Opening Balance		To Honorarium	11300.00
		To Puratattva	47787.50
Cash in hand	5016.62	To Conference Expenses	8752.30
Cash at Bank	11417.08	To Payment to D.D.A.	23292.50
By Grant-in-Aid Received from National Museum	200000.00	To Printing and Stationery	1638.00
		To Conveyance	302.00
By Receipt from Assam Museum	50000.00	To Audit Fees (Previous Year)	2000.00
By Grant-in-Aid Received from I.C.H.R.	9500.00	To Bank Charges	129.00
By Receipt for Vedic Cassette	7588.00	To Entertainment	457.50
By Sale of Publications	9187.50	To Postage	1012.40
By Membership Fees	3860.00	To Vedio Cassette Expenses	5200.00
By Life Membership Fees	11510.00	To Publication Expenses	8754.00
		To Assam Publication Expenses	58850.00
		To Closing Balances	
		Cash in hand	242.92
		Cash at Bank	138361.08
	308079.20		308079.20

Sd/-
(K.N. Dikshit)
General Secretary

Sd/-
(S.P. Asthana)
Treasurer

For Rajan Sharma & Co
Chartered Accountants

Sd/-
(Rajan Kumar Sharma)
Prop.

M.N. 84457.

Place: New Delhi

Date: 4.10.1991

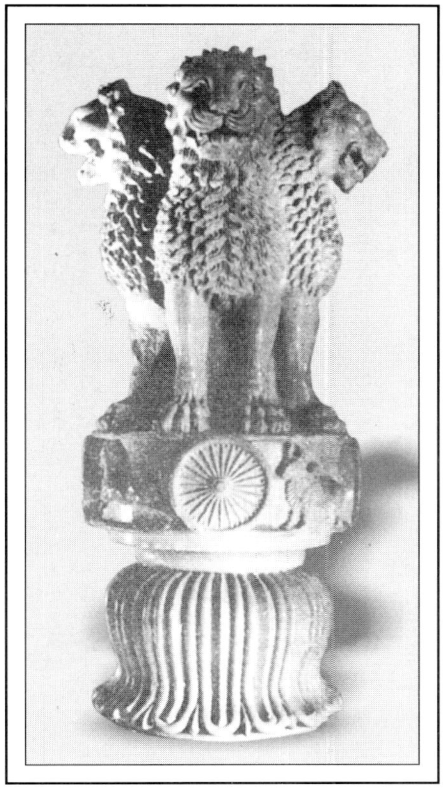

Pl. I. Aśokan Pillar Capital — Sarnath Museum (M.C. Joshi)

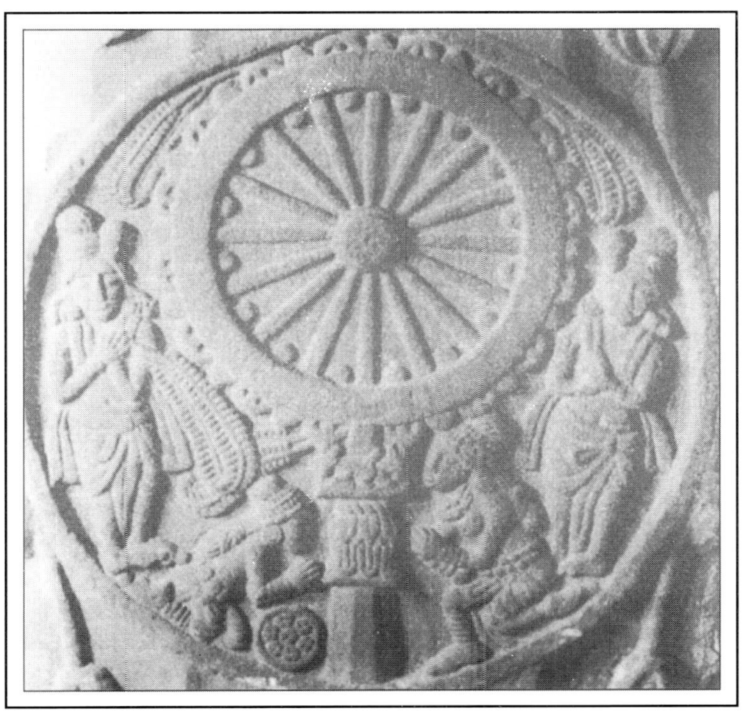

Pl. II. Bharhut relief — Indian Museum (M.C. Joshi)

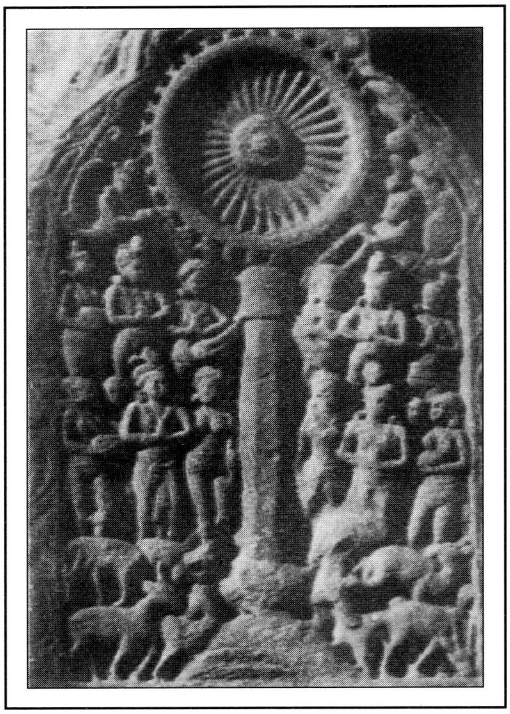

Pl. III. Sanchi relief in southern toraṇa of great stupa (M.C. Joshi)

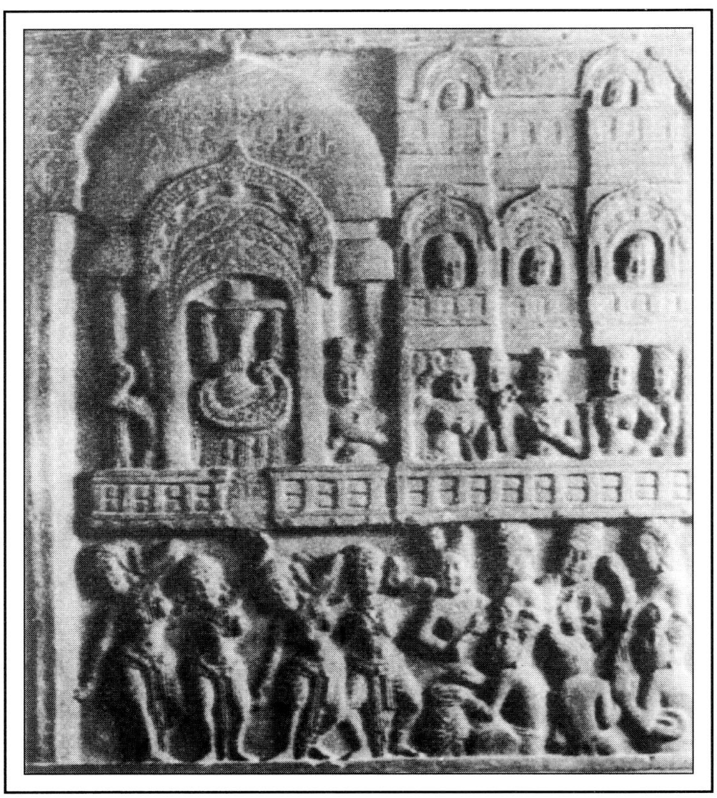

Pl. IV. Bharhut relief — Indian Museum (M.C. Joshi)

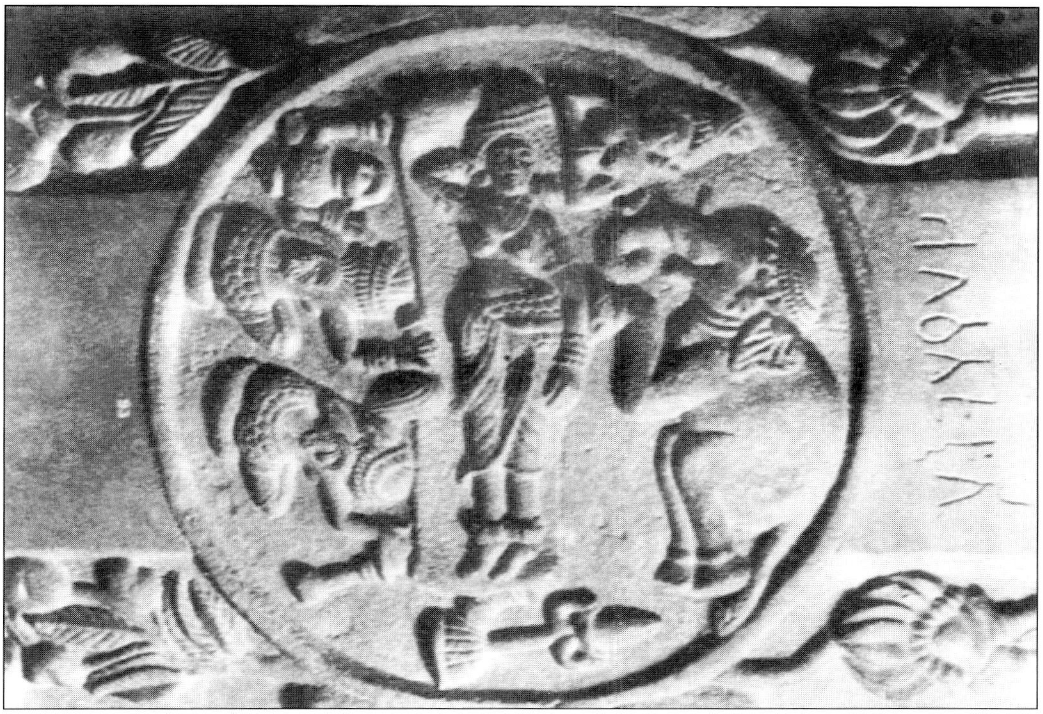

Pl. V. Bharhut relief — Indian Museum (M.C. Joshi)

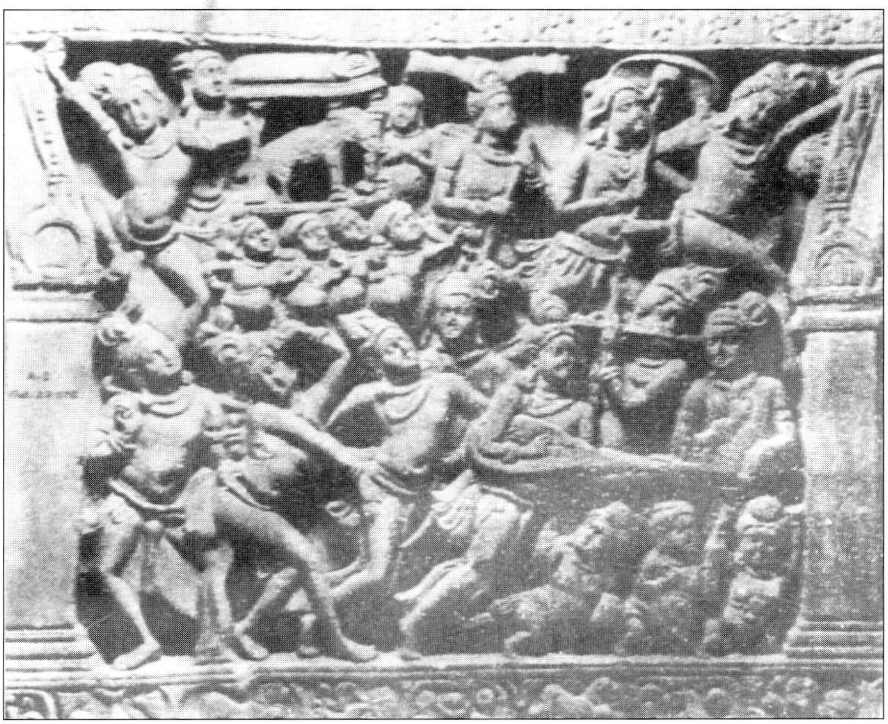

Pl. VI. Amaravati relief — Indian Museum (M.C. Joshi)

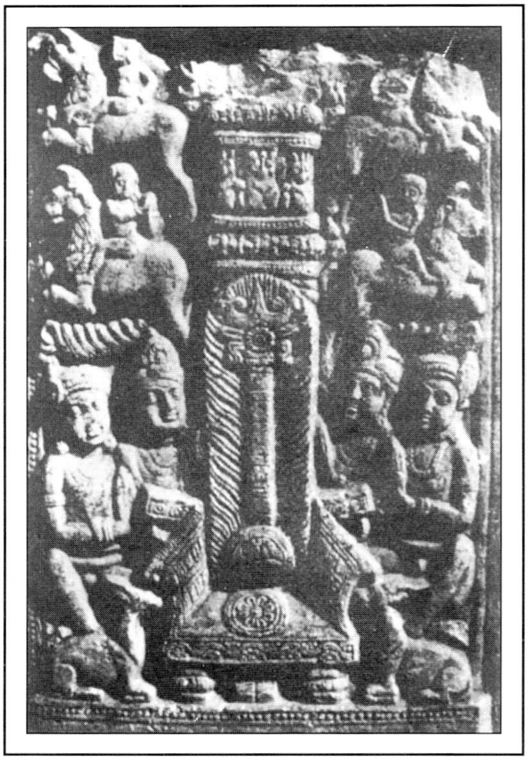

Pl. VII. Amaravati relief (M.C. Joshi)

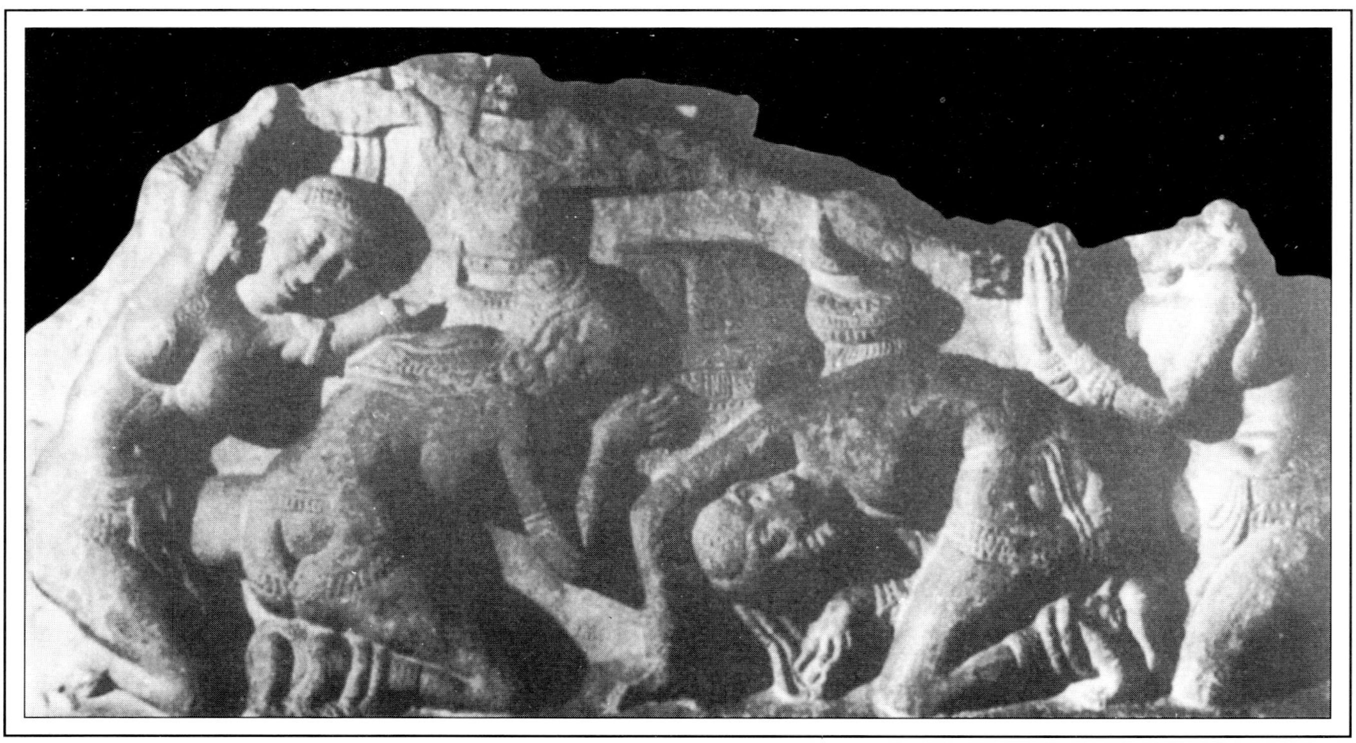

Pl. VIII. Amaravati relief (M.C. Joshi)

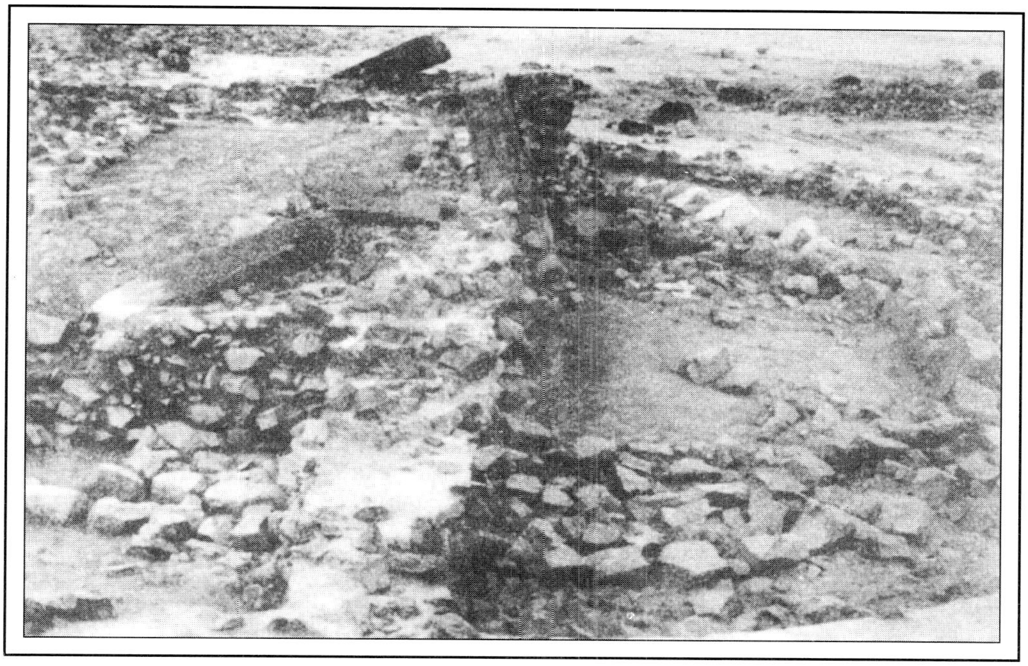

Pl. IX. Megalith, F.I. Karkabhat (A.K. Sharma)

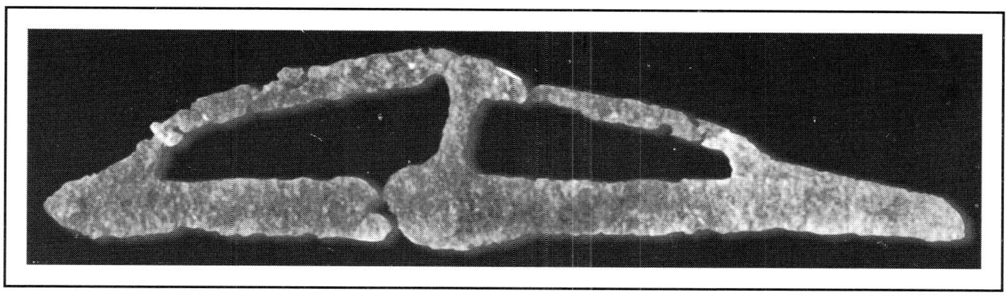

Pl. X. Iron hoe, Karkabhat (A.K. Sharma)

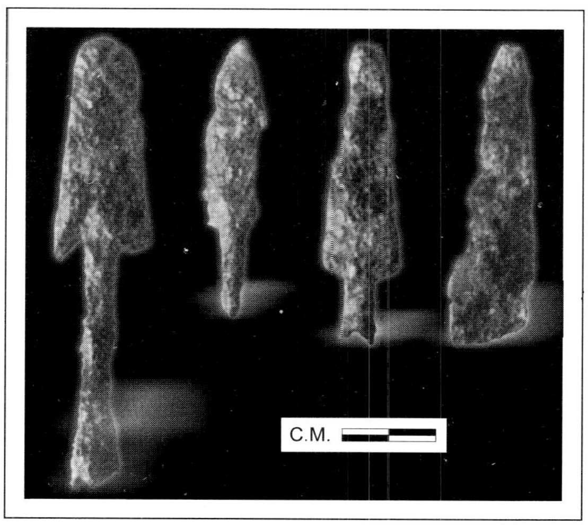

Pl. XI. Iron arrowheads, Karkabhat (A.K. Sharma)

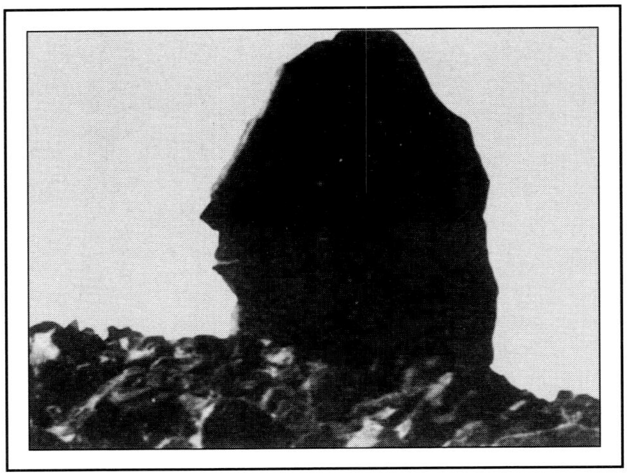

Pl. XII. Menhir, Karkabhat (A.K. Sharma)

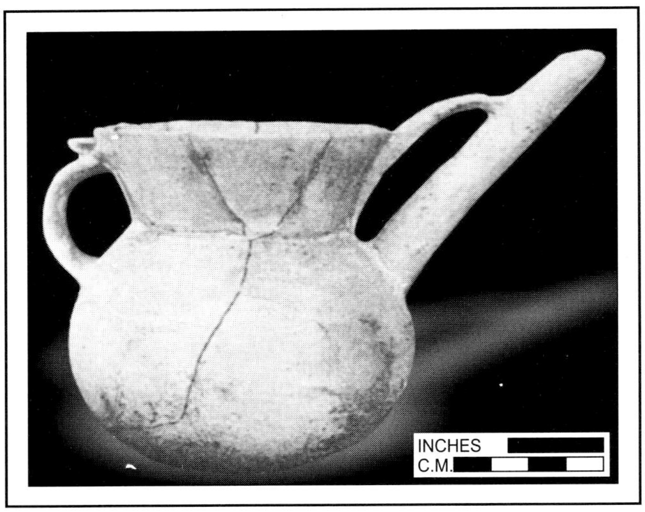

Pl. XIII. Spouted Vessel, Malari (Vinod Nautial *et al.*)

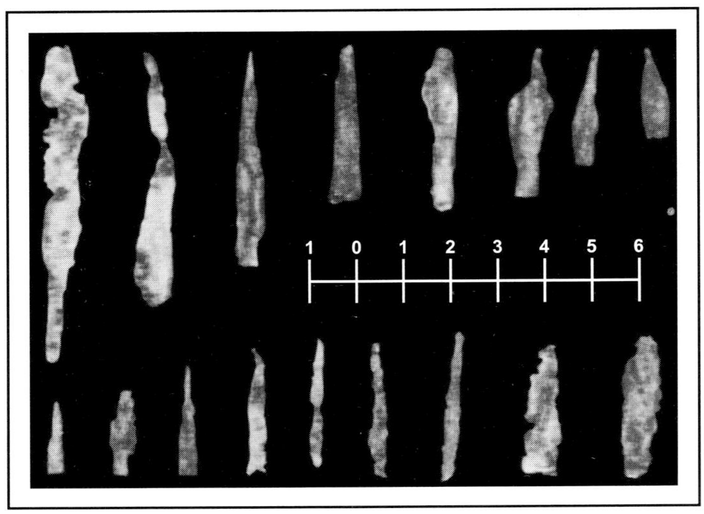

Pl. XIV. Wooden iron implements, Malari (Vinod Nautial *et al.*)

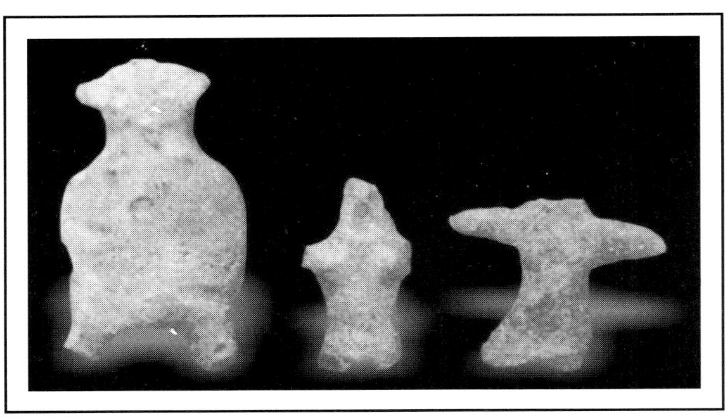

Pl. XV. Archaic terracotta figurines, Siswania (B.R. Mani)

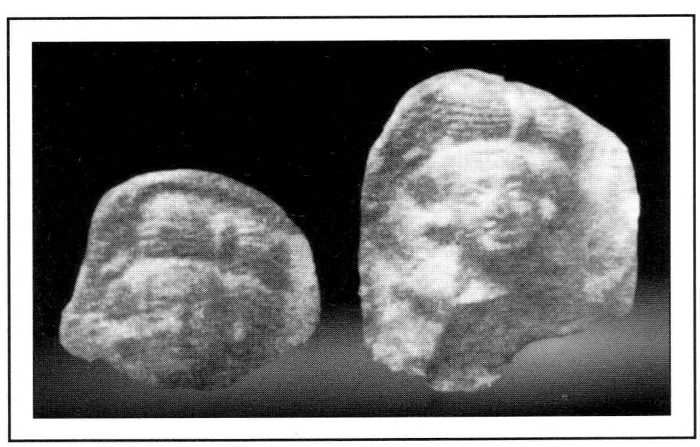

Pl. XVI. Śuṅga terracotta figurines, Siswania (B.R. Mani)

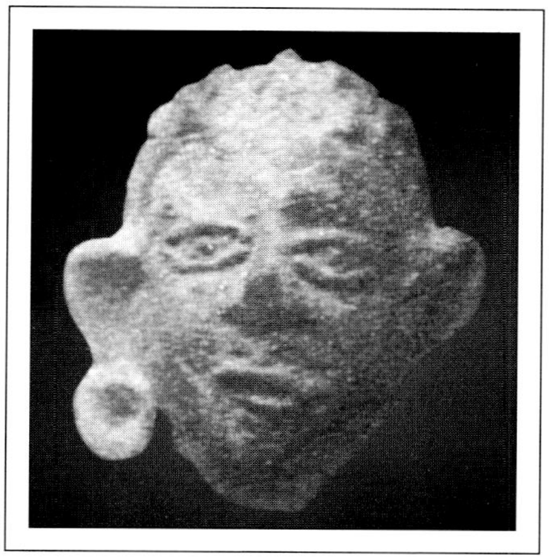

Pl. XVII.

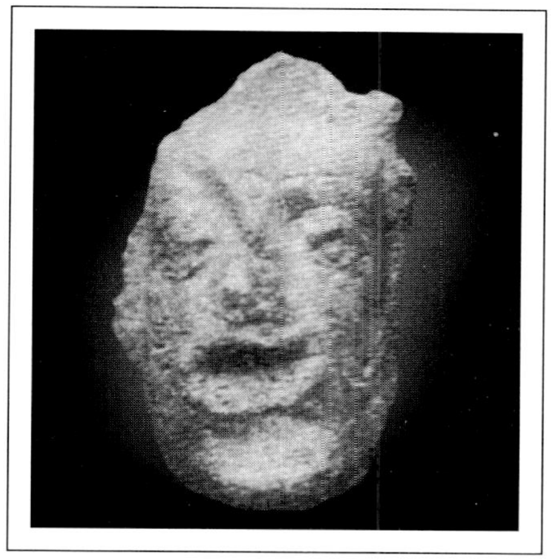

Pl. XVIII.

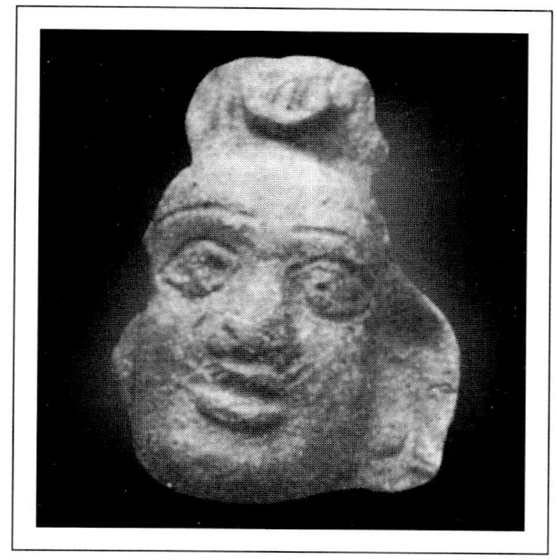

Pl. XIX.

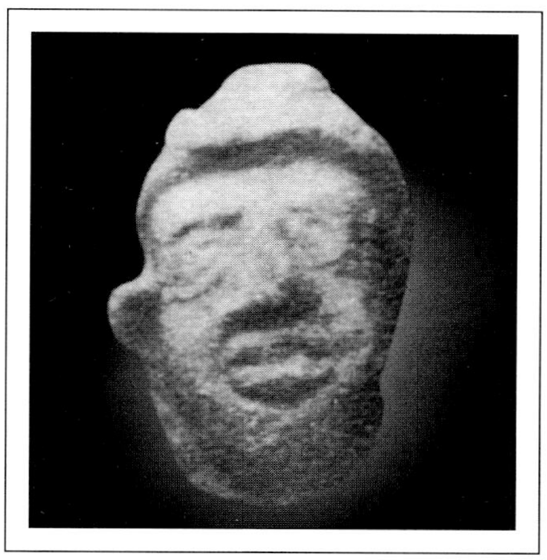

Pl. XX.

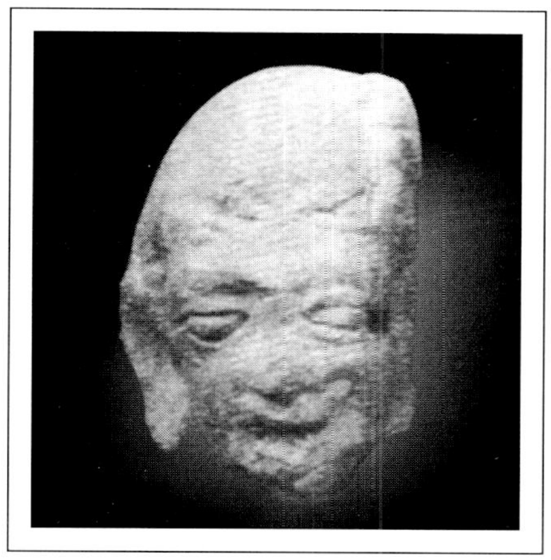

Pl. XXI.

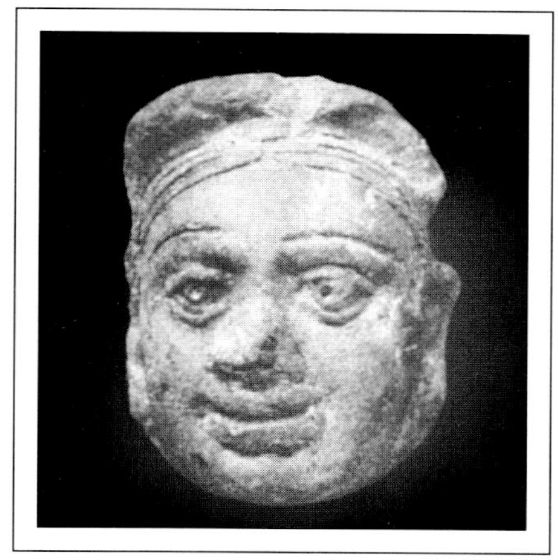

Pl. XXII.

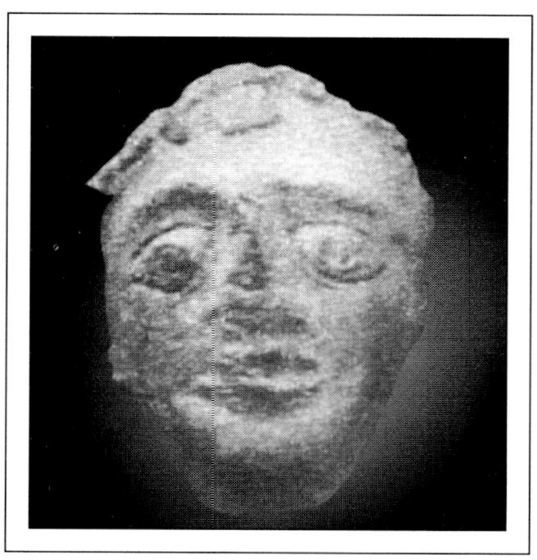

Pl. XXIII.

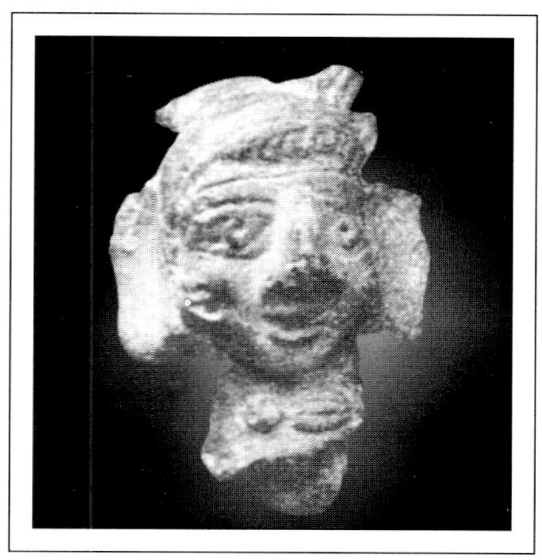

Pl. XXIV.

Plates XVII to XXIV; Kushan terracotta heads, Siswania (B.R. Mani)

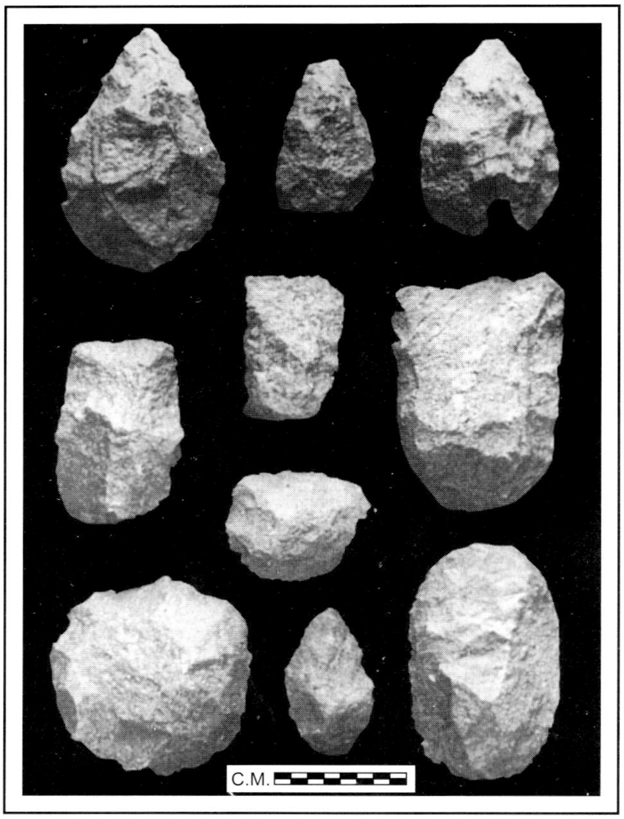

Pl. XXV. Late Acheulian tools, Anangpur (A.K. Sharma)

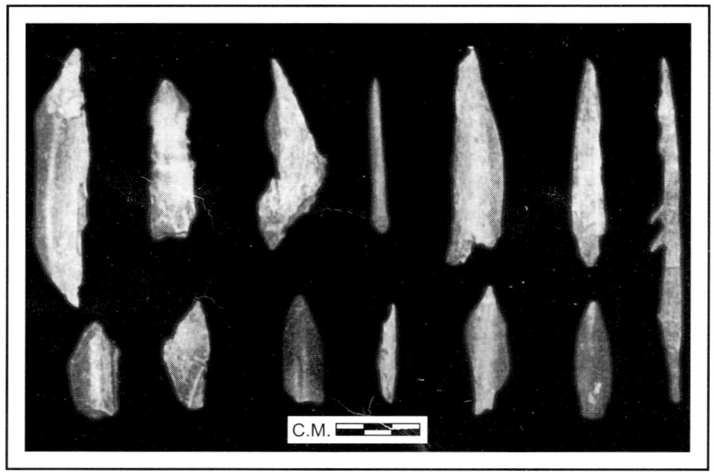

Pl. XXVI. Bone tools, Golabai Sasan (B.K. Sinha)

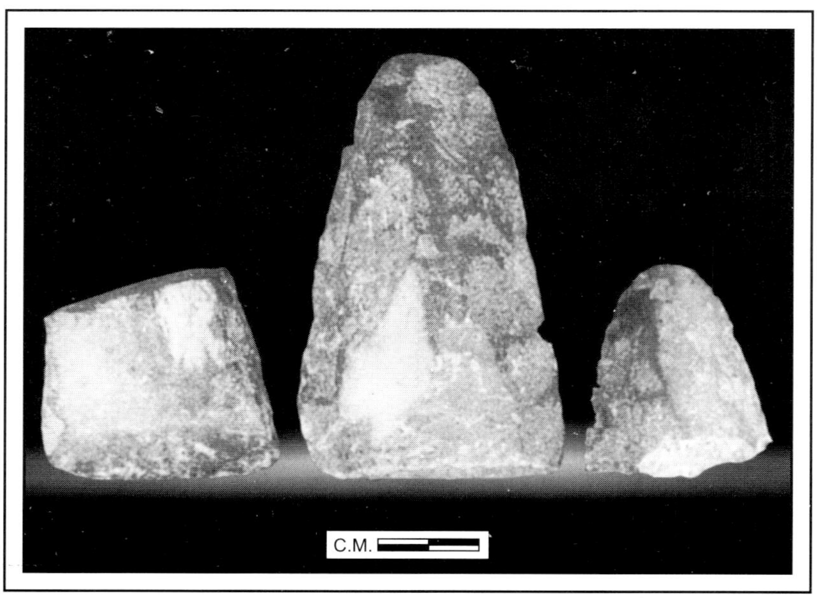

Pl. XXVII. Polished stone tools, Golabai Sasan (B.K. Sinha)

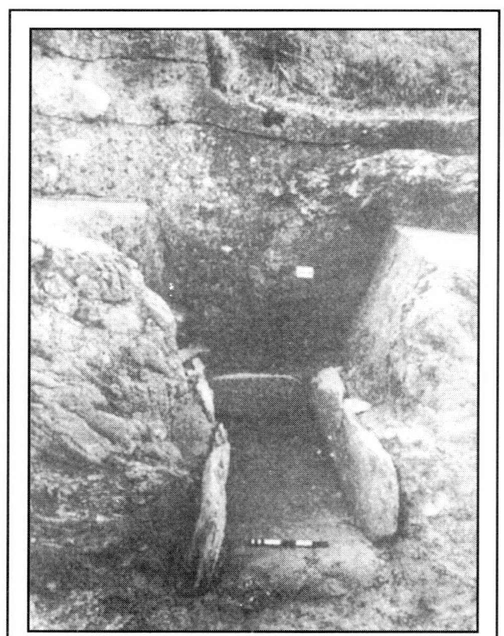

Pl. XXVIII. Excavated remains, Ladyure (A.K. Sharma)

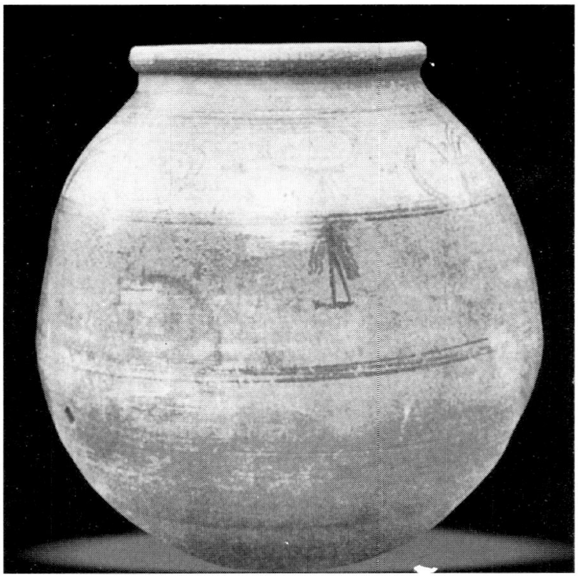

Pl. XXIX. Storage jar, Padri (Vasant Shinde)

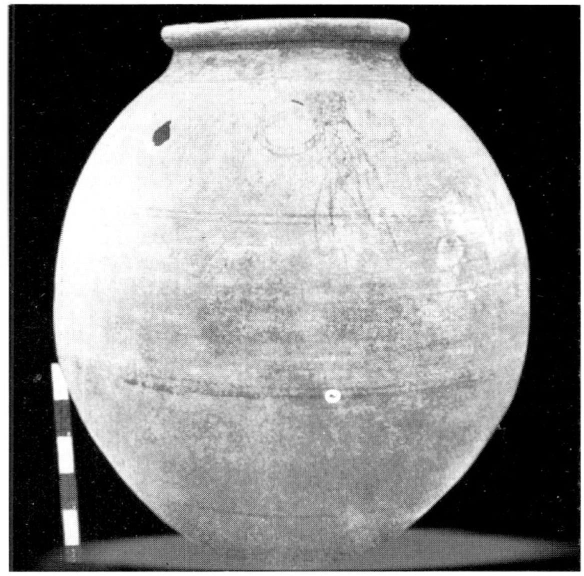

Pl. XXX. Storage jar, Padri (Vasant Shinde)

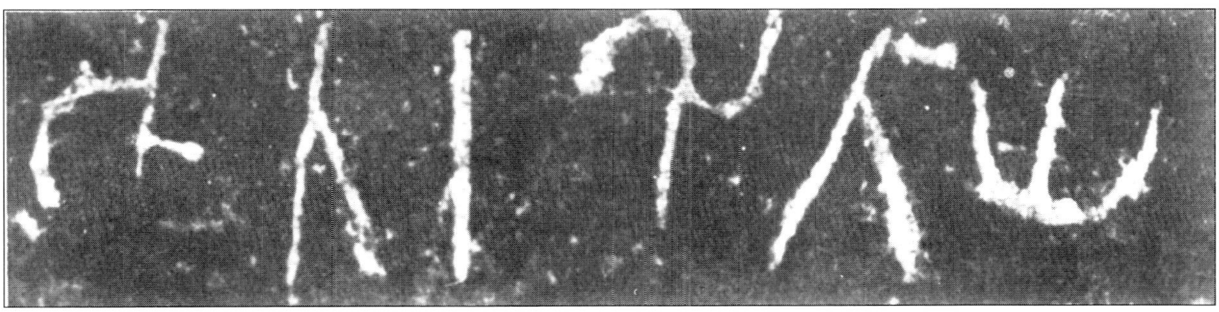

Pl. XXXI. Pitalkhora inscription (S.K. Mitra)

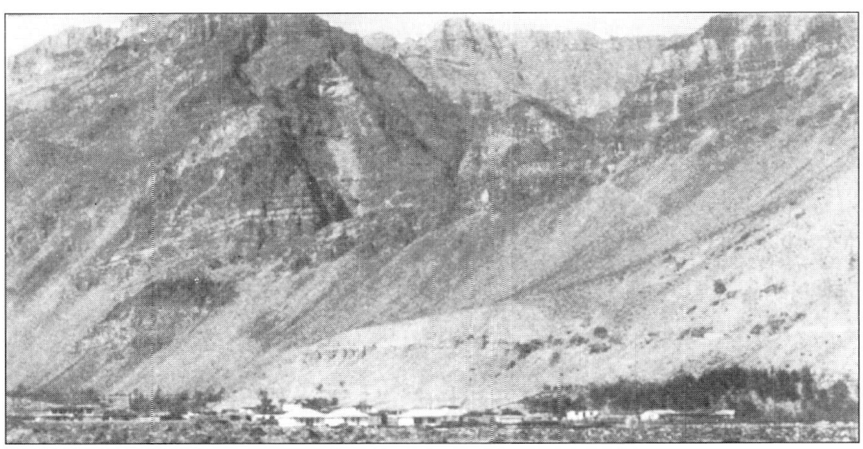

Pl. XXXII. Tabo — General landscape (A.K. Sinha)

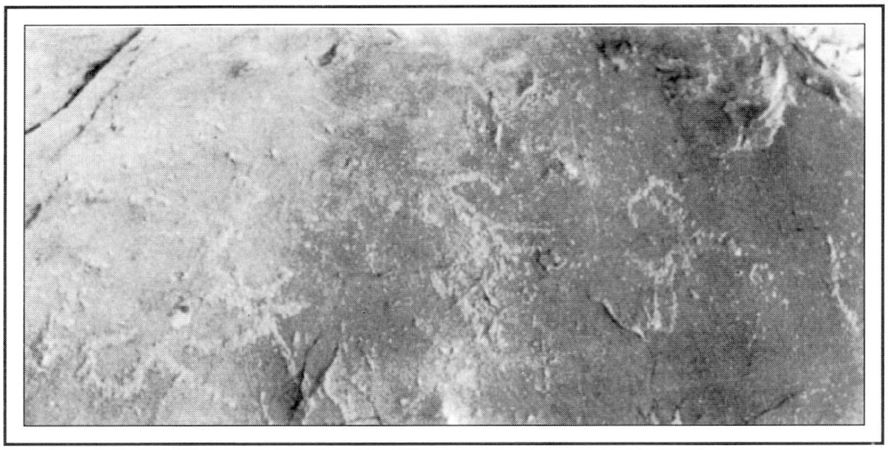

Pl. XXXIII. Rock engravings — Tabo (A.K. Sinha)

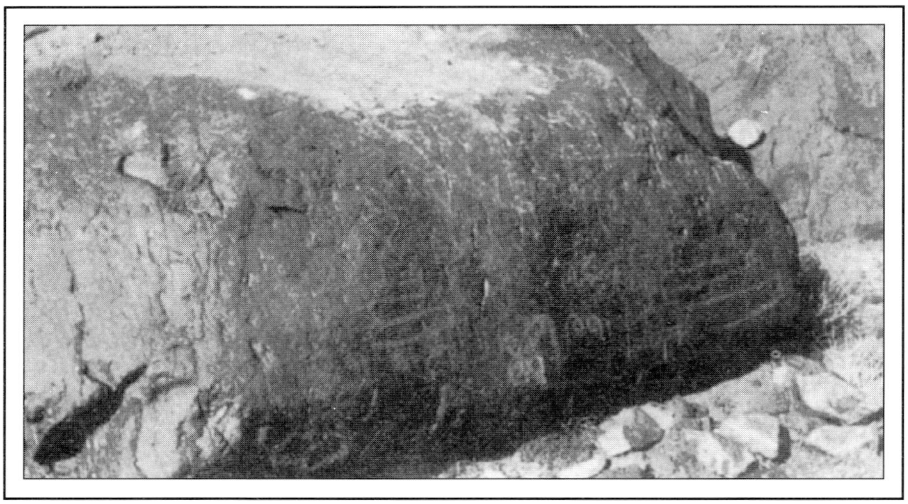

Pl. XXXIV. Rock engravings — Tabo (A.K. Sinha)

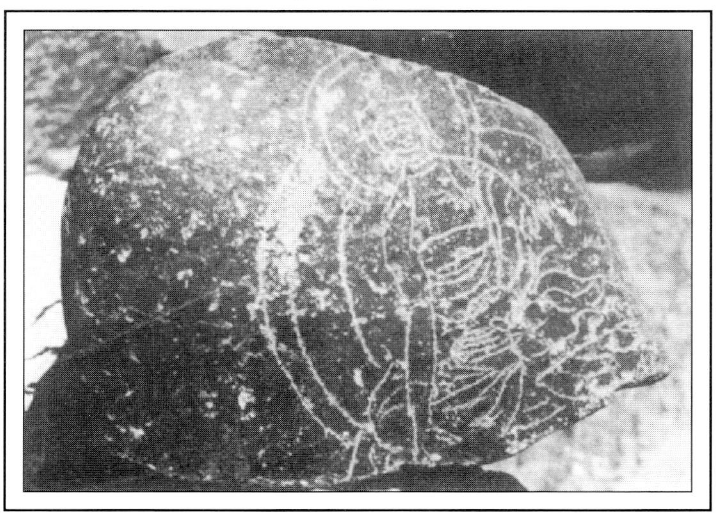

Pl. XXXV. Rock engravings — Tabo (A.K. Sinha)